ARE YOU WATCHING
TRYING TO MAINTAIN A HEALTHY LIFESTYLE?

COOK WITH CONFIDENCE WITH
CORINNE T. NETZER'S
**COMPLETE BOOK OF FOOD COUNTS
COOKBOOK SERIES**
DON'T MISS . . .

POTAGE PARMENTIER

A relative of vichyssoise made with chicken stock, it's just as elegant but it's served hot . . . and without the cream. 130 calories; 3.5 grams protein; 17.5 grams carbohydrates; 4.9 grams fat; 6.3 milligrams cholesterol; 90 milligrams sodium

WONDERFUL HASH

An interesting starter for a meal, this dish, made with leftovers, makes even guests exclaim, "Wonderful!" 105 calories; 11.0 grams protein; 9.5 grams carbohydrates; 2.7 grams fat; 27.4 milligrams cholesterol; 75 milligrams sodium

CHICKEN TOSS WITH SPINACH PASTA AND DRIED TOMATOES

This salad is as colorful as it is delicious—creamy white chicken, emerald green pasta, and burgundy-red tomatoes. 215 calories; 12.0 grams protein; 31.0 grams carbohydrates; 5.0 grams fat; 28.5 milligrams cholesterol; 50 milligrams sodium

100 LOW FAT
CHICKEN
AND TURKEY
RECIPES

THE COMPLETE BOOK OF
FOOD COUNTS COOKBOOK SERIES

100 LOW FAT CHICKEN AND TURKEY RECIPES

Corinne T. Netzer

A Dell Book

Published by
Dell Publishing
a division of
Bantam Doubleday Dell Publishing Group, Inc.
1540 Broadway
New York, New York 10036

ISBN: 0-440-22346-6

Printed in the United States of America

Published simultaneously in Canada

April 1997

10   9   8   7   6   5   4   3   2   1

OPM

CONTENTS

INTRODUCTION

Delicious! Delicious! Delicious! This is one of six books that comprise my Complete Book of Food Counts Cookbook Series—which also includes *100 Low Fat Pasta and Grain Recipes, 100 Low Fat Fish and Shellfish Recipes, 100 Low Fat Vegetable and Legume Recipes, 100 Low Fat Soup and Stew Recipes,* and *100 Low Fat Small Meal and Salad Recipes.* And all the recipes are *delicious*!

We are all aware of the need to reduce the fat in our diets, and ordinarily this would mean a sacrifice in taste. How many of us have had the misfortune to sample some very forgettable low fat dishes, where the overriding concern was only the fat content? It is my belief that no matter how "good" something is for you, you will not continue to eat it if it doesn't *taste* good, and this will almost certainly defeat your diet.

Every recipe in this book has been tested and sampled so that each dish is as good tasting as it is good for you. Low fat ingredients were not used automatically because they might fit or seemed right. Everything was tried out, because not all ingredients are interchangeable—and what might make sense in theory or at the drawing board may not please the palate.

Here you will find wonderful dishes—both plain and fancy—simple fare to eat and serve on a daily basis, and simply elegant fare that you will be proud to serve on any special occasion. Attention has been paid to the use of herbs and spices, but all the ingredients in these recipes can be found either in your cupboard or in the supermarket.

Good eating!

CTN

STOCKS, STUFFINGS, AND SAUCES FOR CHICKEN AND TURKEY

LOW FAT CHICKEN STOCK

This is a lovely, mild-flavored stock that can be used for just about any purpose, and a quick glance through these pages will show you how versatile it is! Cook it down (by about one-quarter), and it's a wonderful and welcome consommé—try it with cooked noodles, pasta, or rice.

For future-use convenience, freeze the stock in ice cube trays (remove when frozen and place in plastic bag) or in one-cup portions to use in recipes; it will keep for about a month. Or refrigerate the stock for up to one week.

  2 pounds chicken parts (backs, wings, necks)
 10 cups water
  $1/2$ cup dry white wine, optional
  1 large onion, quartered
  2 large carrots, coarsely chopped
  2 large stalks celery, with tops, coarsely chopped
  1 bay leaf
  $1/2$ teaspoon whole peppercorns
  8 sprigs fresh parsley
    Salt to taste

1. Combine all ingredients in a soup pot and bring to a boil. Cover, reduce heat to very low and simmer for about 3 hours, skimming stock as necessary. Remove from heat and let cool to room temperature.

2. Strain stock and discard solids or reserve for other use.

3. Cover and refrigerate stock for at least 4 hours or until very well chilled.

4. Skim off hardened surface fat and discard. Stock is ready to be used or may be refrigerated or frozen in airtight containers for later use.

MAKES ABOUT 8 CUPS

Per 1 cup serving: 25 calories; 1.0 gram protein; 2.0 grams carbohydrates; 1.5 grams fat; 5 milligrams cholesterol; 65 milligrams sodium (without salting).

LOW FAT TURKEY-HERB STOCK

Here's one of the best ways to dispose of the holiday turkey carcass (for another way, see my Day-After-Thanksgiving Soup on page 45). This is also an ideal way to cook up the turkey (or chicken) meat you want for salads, sandwiches, stews, and numerous other purposes.

If you want the meat, substitute a whole small or half turkey breast (or a whole chicken cut in half) for the carcass; remove it from the stock before refrigerating it. When the turkey has cooled, remove and discard the skin and grizzle—the meat, which will literally fall off the bones, is ready to use.

   1 turkey carcass or 2 pounds turkey parts (necks, backs, wings) and giblets, cut in pieces
  10 cups water
   1 cup dry red wine
   4 large shallots, coarsely chopped
   1 large clove garlic, coarsely chopped
   1 carrot, coarsely chopped
   1 large stalk celery, with top, coarsely chopped
   1 bay leaf
   6 sprigs parsley
 1/2 teaspoon whole peppercorns
 1/4 teaspoon each: dried thyme, basil, rosemary, sage
      Salt to taste

   1. Combine all ingredients in a soup pot or Dutch oven and bring to a boil. Reduce heat to very low,

cover, and let simmer for 3 hours. Skim stock as necessary. Remove from heat and let cool to room temperature.

2. Remove carcass and discard, or set aside turkey meat to be used for another purpose. Strain stock and discard solids or reserve for other use.

3. Cover and refrigerate stock for at least 4 hours or until very well chilled.

4. Skim off hardened surface fat and discard. Stock is ready to be used or may be refrigerated or frozen in airtight containers for future use.

MAKES ABOUT 8 CUPS

Per 1 cup serving: 30 calories; 1.0 gram protein; 2.0 grams carbohydrates; 2.0 grams fat; 5 milligrams cholesterol; 75 milligrams sodium (without salting).

STUFFINGS FOR CHICKEN AND TURKEY

Whether it's a holiday turkey or an everyday chicken, stuffing is a perfect companion to roasted poultry. Stuffing also complements boiled, broiled, braised, or barbecued birds.

Although the four fabulous recipes that follow will fill a 12- to 14-pound turkey, I prefer cooking the stuffing outside and alongside the bird—that way, it's much easier to serve and it won't pick up the fats from the fowl. To cook the stuffing separately, transfer it to a 9×13-inch nonstick baking pan or an ovenproof casserole lightly coated with vegetable spray and place in oven 45 minutes to 1 hour before bird is done. Add a little stock or water if too much liquid evaporates during baking.

If you want to stuff the turkey be sure to do it *just* before roasting to avoid harmful bacteria that can develop when the stuffing sits inside a warm bird.

HERBED BREAD STUFFING WITH TURKEY SAUSAGE AND APPLES

If you want to prepare this stuffing in advance and refrigerate it overnight, don't add the stock until an hour or so before you're ready to put it in the oven (or the bird) or the stuffing will get soggy.

$1^1/2$ tablespoons vegetable oil
1 onion, diced
$1/4$ pound sweet Italian turkey sausage, casings removed
1 cup coarsely chopped mushrooms, wiped clean
4 slices day-old whole wheat or white bread, cut into $1/2$-inch cubes
1 tablespoon chopped fresh parsley or $1/2$ tablespoon dried
1 teaspoon dried sage
$1/2$ teaspoon each: dried thyme, rosemary, and savory
Salt and freshly ground pepper to taste
1 large tart apple, peeled, cored, and cubed
2 teaspoons fresh lemon juice
$1^1/2$ cups Low Fat Chicken Stock (page 3) or canned low sodium broth

1. Heat oil in a large, deep skillet. Add onion and cook over medium heat, stirring, for 2 minutes. Add turkey sausage to skillet and cook, stirring frequently, for 5 minutes. Add mushrooms, reduce heat to low, and cook for an additional 5 minutes or until turkey sausage is cooked through. Remove from heat.

2. Add all remaining ingredients to skillet, except stock or broth, and mix well. Pour broth over all and stir to combine; if mixture is too dry, add additional broth.

3. Stuff turkey loosely just before roasting, or transfer mixture to a baking pan or an ovenproof casserole coated with cooking spray and place in oven 45 minutes to 1 hour before bird is done (if too much liquid evaporates while baking, add additional stock or water).

MAKES ABOUT 6 CUPS

Per ½ cup serving: 75 calories; 3.0 grams protein; 8.5 grams carbohydrates; 3.5 grams fat; 10 milligrams cholesterol; 110 milligrams sodium (without salting).

WILD RICE AND DRIED
TOMATO STUFFING

Use this delicious stuffing with turkey, chicken, duck, or any wild fowl. It can also stand on its own, with a side of cranberry sauce or relish.

1 1/2 tablespoons vegetable or peanut oil
1 large onion, chopped
2 large stalks celery, chopped
2 cloves garlic, minced
1 cup wild rice
1/2 cup brown rice
2 cups Low Fat Turkey-Herb Stock (page 5), Low Fat Chicken Stock (page 3), or canned low sodium chicken broth
2 cups water
3/4 cup no-salt-added dried tomatoes
1/4 cup chopped fresh basil or parsley or 2 tablespoons dried
Salt and freshly ground pepper to taste

1. Heat oil in a soup pot or Dutch oven. Add onion and celery and cook over medium-high heat, stirring frequently, for 2 minutes. Stir in garlic.

2. Add wild and brown rice to pot and stir briefly to coat grains. Add stock and water and bring to a boil. Reduce heat to low, cover, and simmer for 30 minutes.

3. Meanwhile cover dried tomatoes with very hot

water and let stand until softened. Drain and finely dice.

4. Stir diced tomatoes, basil, and salt and pepper into rice and continue cooking, covered, for an additional 15 minutes or until rice is tender but still chewy; add additional water if too much liquid has evaporated. Remove from heat and let stand, covered, for 10 minutes.

5. Drain any excess liquid if necessary and fluff rice with a fork. Stuff turkey loosely just before roasting, or transfer mixture to a baking pan or an ovenproof casserole coated with cooking spray and place in oven about 45 minutes before bird is done (if too much liquid evaporates while baking, add additional stock or water).

MAKES ABOUT 6 CUPS
Per ½ cup serving: 120 calories; 3.5 grams protein; 21.5 grams carbohydrates; 2.3 grams fat; 1 milligram cholesterol; 30 milligrams sodium (without salting).

BULGUR STUFFING WITH CRANBERRIES AND CHESTNUTS

Fiber-rich and filled with nutrients, this stuffing helps make a holiday dinner extra-special.

1/2 cup Burgundy or other full-bodied red wine
1/4 cup water
2 tablespoons sugar
1 1/2 cups fresh cranberries, rinsed and picked over
1 1/2 tablespoons vegetable or peanut oil
6 shallots, coarsely chopped
1 1/2 cups bulgur
3 cups Low Fat Chicken Stock (page 3) or canned low sodium broth
1/2 pound chestnuts (about 16), roasted, shelled, peeled, and coarsely chopped
1 teaspoon each: dried thyme, mint, and sage
Salt and freshly ground pepper to taste

1. Combine wine, water, and sugar in a large saucepan and bring to a boil. Add cranberries and cook for 2 to 3 minutes or until cranberries have just popped. Set aside to cool.

2. Heat oil in a soup pot or Dutch oven. Add shallots and cook over medium heat, stirring frequently, for about 5 minutes or until shallots are lightly browned. Add bulgur and stir to combine.

3. Using a slotted spoon, transfer cranberries and 1 tablespoon cooking liquid to bulgur mixture (you can

reserve remaining cooking liquid, if any, to baste the bird). Add all remaining ingredients, toss lightly to combine, and simmer over low heat, partially covered, for about 30 minutes or until liquid is absorbed and bulgur is tender. Taste and correct seasonings, if necessary.

4. Stuff turkey loosely just before roasting, or transfer mixture to a baking pan or an ovenproof casserole coated with cooking spray and place in oven about 45 minutes before bird is done (if too much liquid evaporates while baking, add additional stock or water).

MAKES ABOUT 6 CUPS

Per ½ cup serving: 135 calories; 3.0 grams protein; 25.5 grams carbohydrates; 2.5 grams fat; 1 milligram cholesterol; 25 milligrams sodium (without salting).

POTATO, LEEK, AND MUSHROOM STUFFING

If you prefer potatoes to stuffing, now you can have both! This dish appeals to just about everyone, and it makes a tasty side dish for any meat, fish, or poultry entrée.

2 medium potatoes, peeled and cubed
1 tablespoon vegetable oil
2 leeks, white and tender greens, rinsed and chopped
1 stalk celery, diced
2 cups sliced mushrooms
Salt and freshly ground pepper to taste
1/4 cup dry white wine
1/4 cup plus 1 tablespoon chopped fresh dill weed
2 slices day-old whole wheat or white bread, cut into
1/2-inch cubes
1/2 cup Low Fat Turkey-Herb Stock (page 5), Low Fat Chicken Stock (page 3), or canned low sodium chicken broth, approximately

1. Cover potatoes with water in a small saucepan and bring to a boil. Reduce heat slightly and simmer for 15 to 20 minutes or until potatoes are just tender. Drain and set aside.

2. While potatoes cook, heat oil in a large nonstick skillet. Add leeks and celery and cook over medium heat, stirring frequently, for 5 minutes.

3. Add mushrooms and 1/4 cup dill to skillet. Stir in salt, pepper, and wine and bring to a simmer. Reduce

heat to low, cover, and let simmer gently, stirring occasionally, for 10 minutes.

4. Add potato and bread cubes to skillet and stir or toss lightly to combine ingredients.

5. Spoon mixture into a nonstick baking pan or ovenproof casserole coated with cooking spray. Drizzle with stock and sprinkle top with remaining tablespoon dill. Put in oven for 30 minutes before bird is done or bake in preheated 350° F. oven (if too much liquid evaporates while baking, add additional stock or water).

MAKES ABOUT 6 CUPS
Per ½ cup serving: 55 calories; 1.5 grams protein; 9.0 grams carbohydrates; 1.5 grams fat; 0 milligrams cholesterol; 30 milligrams sodium (without salting).

CREAMY SHALLOT SAUCE

This low fat sauce, a creamy blend of shallots, scallions, herbs, and reduced chicken stock, transforms plain poached chicken into something special. It's also the perfect gravy for whipped potatoes, squash, or turnips, and it's a fabulous braising sauce for leeks, celery, or endives.

    2 teaspoons vegetable oil
    4 shallots, coarsely chopped
    2 scallions, white part only, chopped
    ¹/₄ teaspoon dried thyme
    ¹/₄ teaspoon dry mustard
       Salt and freshly ground pepper to taste
    ¹/₄ cup dry white wine
1¹/₂ cups Low Fat Chicken Stock (page 3) or canned low
       sodium broth
    1 tablespoon fine flour
    2 tablespoons low fat sour cream

1. Heat oil in a small nonstick skillet. Add shallots and scallions and cook, stirring frequently, over medium heat for 5 minutes or until golden brown. Add thyme, mustard, and salt and pepper and stir to blend.

2. Add wine and ¹/₂ cup stock to skillet. Raise heat to high and bring to a boil. Stir for about 1 minute, then remove from heat.

3. In a small saucepan, bring remaining 1 cup of stock to a boil. Reduce heat slightly and let simmer,

uncovered, until reduced by about half. Reduce heat to low.

4. While stock simmers, transfer shallots with contents of skillet to a food processor and process until smoothly blended. Transfer shallot mixture to saucepan with stock and stir until ingredients are thoroughly combined.

5. Mix flour and sour cream in a small bowl and stir into shallot-stock mixture. Cook over very low heat, stirring constantly, until sauce is smoothly blended, thickened, and just simmering.

MAKES ABOUT 1¹/₂ CUPS

Per ¹/₄ cup serving: 40 calories; 1.0 gram protein; 4.0 grams carbohydrates; 2.5 grams fat; 3 milligrams cholesterol; 25 milligrams sodium (without salting).

CRANBERRY-LEMON SAUCE AND GLAZE

Brush this smooth, sweet-and-tart glaze over skinless chicken or turkey during broiling or roasting, and offer it as a side dish sauce as well. To accommodate roasting an 18- to 20-pound turkey, just double the recipe.

If you will not be using the glaze immediately, it can be refrigerated in an airtight container for three or four days. Cook briefly over low heat just before using.

1½ cups fresh cranberries, rinsed and picked over
⅔ cup water
⅓ cup Madeira or port wine
⅓ cup sugar
2 tablespoons fresh lemon juice
1 teaspoon grated lemon zest

1. Combine all ingredients in a medium saucepan and cook over medium-high heat, stirring frequently, for about 3 minutes or until sugar is dissolved and cranberries start to pop. Reduce heat to low and simmer gently for 2 minutes. Remove from heat and let cool slightly.

2. Transfer to a food processor or blender and puree.

MAKES ABOUT 2 CUPS
Per ¼ cup serving: 45 calories; .1 gram protein; 11.5 grams carbohydrates; trace fat; 0 milligrams cholesterol; 1 milligram sodium (without salting).

SPICED MARINADE AND DIPPING SAUCE

However you prepare poultry, try this all-purpose sauce as a marinade, basting, and/or dipping sauce when you want to add zing to an otherwise boring presentation.

2 shallots, quartered
2 cloves garlic, quartered
2 teaspoons minced fresh peeled ginger
2 tablespoons chopped fresh cilantro, optional
1/2 teaspoon dried cumin
1/2 cup rice or white wine vinegar
1/4 cup water
1 tablespoon low sodium soy sauce
1/4 teaspoon hot sesame or chili oil, optional
2 tablespoons peanut oil

1. Combine all ingredients, except peanut oil, in a food processor and process until well blended. With processor running, add oil in a slow steady stream.

2. Transfer to a small bowl and let stand for at least 30 minutes before using, to allow flavors to blend.

MAKES ABOUT 1 CUP
Per 2 tablespoon serving: 20 calories; .5 gram protein; 2.0 grams carbohydrates; 1.2 grams fat; 0 milligrams cholesterol; 75 milligrams sodium (without salting).

SOUPS AND
CHOWDERS

OLD-FASHIONED
CHICKEN NOODLE SOUP

After all the jokes that have been made about chicken soup, it turns out that there is some scientific fact behind the theory that this soup is a fine restorative when you have a cold. Sick or well, chicken soup is delicious, and because it often brings back fond memories of family it's also a comfort food.

I prepare the soup a day before I plan to serve it, so that I can skim off the fat that rises to the top after it has been refrigerated.

 1 2½-pound chicken, whole or halved
 2 quarts water
 ½ cup dry white wine, optional
 1 large onion, halved
 2 cloves garlic, halved
 4 stalks celery, halved
 2 carrots, halved
 1 turnip, quartered
   Herb bouquet: 5 sprigs fresh parsley, 5 sprigs dill,
      and 1 bay leaf, tied together
 8 peppercorns
   Salt to taste
1½ cups cooked thin egg noodles
 1 tablespoon chopped fresh parsley

1. Combine all ingredients except salt, noodles, and chopped parsley in a soup pot and bring to a simmer.

Cover and cook, skimming off foam occasionally, for about 2 hours or until chicken is tender. Remove pot from heat and allow soup to cool for about 20 minutes.

2. Using a slotted spoon, remove chicken from soup. Place in covered bowl or wrap in foil and refrigerate.

3. Strain soup, discarding all solids, and refrigerate overnight or until well chilled.

4. The following day or when you're ready to serve the soup, skim fat that has risen to the surface. Heat soup to a simmer.

5. Remove skin, bones, and gristle from the chicken and discard. Cut chicken meat into serving pieces and add to the soup. Add salt to taste and continue simmering until ingredients are heated through.

6. Spoon noodles into heated soup bowls and ladle hot soup over noodles. Chicken may be served with the soup or as a second course. Garnish with parsley and serve hot.

SERVES 6
Per serving: 200 calories; 22.5 grams protein; 20.0 grams carbohydrates; 3.6 grams fat; 77 milligrams cholesterol; 130 milligrams sodium (without salting).

CHICKEN AND ESCAROLE SOUP

Chicory and escarole are often confused with one another, or are referred to by different names in different localities. I happen to love both of these slightly bitter-tasting greens and use them interchangeably in salads and soups.

For the record, chicory forms a loose bunch of ragged-edged leaves on long stems while escarole has loose, elongated heads and broad wavy leaves with smooth edges. Escarole is also milder-tasting than chicory.

1/2 chicken breast (about 1/2 pound), skin and fat
    removed
1 small onion, halved
2 cloves garlic, halved
2 stalks celery, halved
1 carrot, halved
1/4 cup coarsely chopped fresh parsley
4 cups Low Fat Chicken Stock (page 3) or canned low
    sodium broth
1 cup water
  Salt and freshly ground pepper to taste
1 small head escarole

1. Place chicken in a soup pot. Add all remaining ingredients, except escarole. Bring to a simmer, cover, and cook for about 45 minutes or until chicken is tender.

2. While chicken cooks, prepare escarole by discard-

ing tough outer leaves, and separating remaining escarole into leaves. Cut leaves into 1-inch strips and set aside.

3. Using a slotted spoon, remove chicken from pot and let stand until cool enough to handle. Strain soup, discarding all vegetables, and return to pot.

4. When chicken has cooled, remove meat from bones, cut into bite-size pieces and add to soup. Add escarole and bring soup to a simmer. Cook for 3 minutes. Taste and correct seasoning, if necessary, before serving in heated bowls.

SERVES 4

Per serving: 125 calories; 15.5 grams protein; 10.5 grams carbohydrates; 2.7 grams fat; 37 milligrams cholesterol; 150 milligrams sodium (without salting).

CRANBERRY BEANS AND SMOKED CHICKEN CHOWDER

Fresh cranberry beans with their cream and rosy markings have a wonderful flavor but, unfortunately, they're not always available. Substitute a cup of cooked great northern beans if you can't find cranberry beans.

    1 pound unshelled fresh cranberry beans
    1 teaspoon olive oil
    2 cloves garlic, pressed
    1 tablespoon chopped fresh Italian parsley
    2 stalks celery, thinly sliced
    1 small red bell pepper, chopped
    4 cups Low Fat Chicken Stock (page 3) or canned low
        sodium broth
    1 cup water
    1/4 teaspoon hot red pepper flakes or to taste
        Salt to taste
    1/4 pound sliced smoked chicken breast, shredded
    2 plum tomatoes, diced

1. Shell cranberry beans and set aside.

2. Heat oil in a soup pot. Add garlic and cook, stirring, for 1 minute. Add beans and all remaining ingredients, except chicken and tomatoes. Cover and bring to a simmer. Cook for 30 to 45 minutes or until beans are tender.

3. Transfer one cup of soup with beans to a food

processor and puree. Return to soup pot and stir to blend with remaining soup.

4. Bring soup to a simmer and stir chicken into soup. Cook until all ingredients are heated through. Ladle into heated bowls, garnish with diced tomato, and serve.

SERVES 4

Per serving: 140 calories; 11.0 grams protein; 17.5 grams carbohydrates; 3.8 grams fat; 20 milligrams cholesterol; 480 milligrams sodium (without salting).

CHICKEN-TOMATO SOUP WITH ORZO

Orzo is a tiny pasta that looks like grains of rice. That, or *acini de pepe*—pasta that resembles peppercorns—go equally well in this soup.

The real secret here is the flavor of the tomatoes: they must be ripe and juicy. If all you can find at your local supermarket are tomatoes that resemble red rocks, put off making this soup.

    5 large ripe tomatoes
    1 small onion, chopped
    ¹/₂ tablespoon olive oil
    4 cups Low Fat Chicken Stock (page 3) or canned low
        sodium broth
    ¹/₄ cup orzo
    1 cup cubed cooked chicken breast
      Salt and freshly ground pepper to taste
    1 tablespoon chopped fresh basil or parsley

1. Peel, seed, and chop 4 of the tomatoes.

2. Heat oil in a soup pot. Add chopped tomatoes and onion, and cook, stirring, until onion is wilted.

3. Transfer tomato-onion mixture to a food processor and puree. Return to soup pot and cook over low heat, stirring, until mixture is reduced to a paste.

4. Add chicken stock gradually, stirring, and bring to a simmer. Cover and cook for 5 minutes. Add orzo and cook for an additional 5 minutes or until pasta is al dente.

5. Peel, seed, and chop remaining tomato.

6. Add chopped tomato, chicken, and salt and pepper to soup pot. Stir to combine and let simmer until ingredients are heated through. Season to taste. Ladle into heated bowls, garnish with chopped basil or parsley, and serve.

SERVES 4

Per serving: 200 calories; 14.5 grams protein; 25.0 grams carbohydrates; 6.1 grams fat; 31 milligrams cholesterol; 110 milligrams sodium (without salting).

CHICKEN CURRY SOUP
WITH APPLE

Since I've cut down on fat, I've become almost obsessive about finding satisfying replacements for those merciless globs. By experimenting with herbs and spices used in the ethnic cuisines of the world, I've not only come up with truly superb low fat recipes but I'm slowly but surely blotting out my yen for grease. Curry, which is widely used in Indian cooking, is one of the tastiest fat-for-flavor swaps.

> 5 cups Low Fat Chicken Stock (page 3) or canned low sodium broth
> 1 carrot, quartered
> 1/2 small fennel bulb, coarsely chopped
> 4 shallots, chopped
> 1/2 tablespoon curry powder
> 1/2 teaspoon ground cardamom
> Pinch ground cumin
> 1 cup shredded cooked chicken
> Salt and freshly ground pepper to taste
> 1 Granny Smith or other tart apple, peeled, cored, and diced

1. Combine stock, carrot, fennel, and shallots in a soup pot and bring to a simmer. Cover and cook about 15 minutes or until vegetables are tender.

2. Using a slotted spoon, transfer vegetables to a food processor. Add 1/2 cup of stock and process until vegetables are pureed. Return mixture to soup pot.

3. Add curry, cardamom, cumin, and chicken to pot. Heat to a simmer, and cook for 3 minutes.

4. Add salt, pepper, and apple and simmer until all ingredients are heated through. Serve hot.

SERVES 4

Per serving: 140 calories; 11.5 grams protein; 15.5 grams carbohydrates; 4.2 grams fat; 33 milligrams cholesterol; 125 milligrams sodium (without salting).

POTAGE PARMENTIER

Here's the soup that's the forerunner of vichyssoise. Many of the ingredients are the same, but Potage Parmentier is served hot, and tastes delicious without the cream.

2 teaspoons olive oil
2 onions, thinly sliced
2 medium potatoes, peeled and cubed
5 cups Low Fat Chicken Stock (page 3) or canned low sodium broth
   Salt and freshly ground pepper to taste
2 tablespoons grated carrot

1. Heat olive oil in a soup pot. Add onions and potatoes, and cook, stirring, over low heat for 2 minutes.

2. Add stock to pot and bring to a simmer. Cover and cook for about 20 minutes or until potatoes are tender.

3. Using a slotted spoon, transfer onion and potatoes to a food processor and process until just smooth. Don't overprocess or potatoes will acquire a pasty texture.

4. Return pureed vegetables to soup pot. Stir and bring to a simmer. Cook for 2 minutes and season to taste.

5. Ladle soup into heated bowls, garnish with grated carrot, and serve.

SERVES 4

Per serving: 130 calories; 3.5 grams protein; 17.5 grams carbohydrates; 4.9 grams fat; 6 milligrams cholesterol; 90 milligrams sodium (without salting).

VEGETABLE AND CHICKEN CHOWDER

"Chowder" describes a thick, rich soup containing chunks of food, whether it's the familiar one containing clams or fish or the robust, soul-stirring kind brimming with vegetables. My Vegetable and Chicken Chowder combines the best of both chowders, producing a delicious, filling, and low fat dish.

Serve it hot with a coarse bread, such as Italian whole wheat or black bread.

6 cups water
1 pound skinless and boneless chicken breasts
    Salt and freshly ground pepper to taste
4 cups Low Fat Chicken Stock (page 3) or canned low sodium broth
2 medium potatoes, peeled and diced
2 small zucchini, coarsely chopped
6 scallions, white and tender greens, chopped
1/4 pound green beans, cut into 2-inch lengths
1 cup shredded cabbage

1. Combine water, chicken breasts, and salt and pepper in a soup pot and bring to a boil. Reduce heat to medium low and simmer, covered, for 45 minutes. Using a slotted spoon, remove chicken breasts from pot and set aside until cool enough to handle.

2. Add potato to liquid in pot. Cover and cook for 10 minutes.

3. Add zucchini and cook for 5 minutes.

4. While potatoes cook, cut chicken breast into bite-size pieces.

5. Add chicken, along with all remaining ingredients and cook, covered, for an additional 5 to 10 minutes or until vegetables are tender. Taste and adjust seasonings, if necessary. Ladle into heated bowls and serve.

SERVES 6

Per serving: 140 calories; 19.5 grams protein; 11.0 grams carbohydrates; 2.3 grams fat; 46 milligrams cholesterol; 100 milligrams sodium (without salting).

LEMON CHICKEN SOUP WITH DILL

Somewhat reminiscent of the Greek soup *Avgolemono,* which has rice and is made from chicken broth, egg yolks, and lemon juice, my luscious soup deletes the yolks and adds fresh dill, which blends beautifully with the chicken and lemon flavors.

4 cups Low Fat Chicken Stock (page 3) or canned low sodium broth
2 cups water
1 small onion, chopped
1/3 cup rice
2 tablespoons fresh chopped dill weed or 1 tablespoon dried
Salt and freshly ground pepper to taste
1/4 cup fresh lemon juice
1 cup diced cooked chicken breast
Fresh dill sprigs for garnish

1. Combine stock, water, onion, rice, dill weed, and salt and pepper in a soup pot. Bring to a boil, then reduce heat to low and simmer, partially covered, for 20 minutes or until rice is tender.

2. Add lemon juice and chicken. Stir and cook, uncovered, for an additional 5 minutes. Ladle into heated bowls and serve garnished with dill sprigs.

Per serving: 150 calories; 12.0 grams protein; 17.5 grams carbohydrates; 3.6 grams fat; 31 milligrams cholesterol; 90 milligrams sodium (without salting).

TURKEY-SQUASH BISQUE

The glorious pale yellow color of this rich-tasting soup reflects the burst of beta-carotene you'll get from the squash and carrot in it. Truly a natural for autumn and winter months.

1 medium butternut squash, peeled, seeded, and diced
1 onion, chopped
1 carrot, sliced
4 cups Low Fat Turkey-Herb Stock (page 5) or canned low sodium chicken broth
1 teaspoon dried thyme
1 bay leaf
    Salt and freshly ground pepper to taste
1 tablespoon vegetable oil
2 tablespoons fine flour
1/2 cup finely diced cooked turkey meat
1/2 cup evaporated low fat milk
2 tablespoons chopped fresh chives

1. Combine squash, onion, carrot, stock, thyme, bay leaf, and salt and pepper in a soup pot. Bring to a boil, then reduce heat to low, cover, and simmer gently for 20 to 30 minutes or until squash is tender.

2. Drain squash and vegetables, reserving liquid and discarding bay leaf. Pour cooking liquid into a bowl but do not wash soup pot. Put squash and vegetables in a food processor and process until smoothly pureed.

3. Heat oil in the soup pot. Whisk in flour over very

low heat. Gradually pour in reserved cooking liquid, whisking constantly. Raise heat to medium high and add pureed squash. Stir constantly over low heat for 1 minute or until well blended. Add turkey and milk and continue to stir until thoroughly blended and heated.

4. Transfer soup into heated bowls, sprinkle with chopped chives, and serve.

SERVES 4
Per serving: 195 calories; 10.5 grams protein; 25.5 grams carbohydrates; 7.1 grams fat; 20 milligrams cholesterol; 130 milligrams sodium (without salting).

LENTIL SOUP WITH
ITALIAN TURKEY SAUSAGE

As this recipe illustrates, your taste buds need not suffer from "fat withdrawal" when you lower your fat intake. Depending on your preference, use either hot or sweet Italian turkey sausage—both are seasoned to taste like the far-fattier pork sausage.

1 teaspoon olive oil
1/4 pound Italian turkey sausage, cut into 1/4-inch rounds
1/4 pound lentils
1 small onion, diced
1 clove garlic, pressed
2 ripe tomatoes, chopped
4 cups Low Fat Chicken Stock (page 3) or canned low
    sodium broth
1/4 teaspoon dried oregano
    Salt and freshly ground pepper to taste

1. Heat oil in a small nonstick skillet. Add sausage and cook over medium heat for about 5 minutes, browning lightly on both sides. Remove sausage from skillet and set aside.

2. Combine all remaining ingredients in a large soup pot and bring to a simmer. Cover, reduce heat to low, and simmer for about 45 minutes or until lentils are tender. (Some lentils absorb a great deal of liquid. Add water, 1/2 cup at a time, if soup seems to be getting too thick.)

3. Transfer one cup of soup with lentils to a food

processor and puree. Return to soup pot and stir to blend with remaining soup.

4. Add sausage slices to soup and return to a simmer. Cook, stirring frequently, for 5 minutes or until thoroughly heated before serving.

SERVES 4

Per serving: 230 calories; 15.0 grams protein; 27.0 grams carbohydrates; 7.6 grams fat; 35 milligrams cholesterol; 270 milligrams sodium (without salting).

TURKEY TORTILLA SOUP
WITH JALAPEÑO PEPPER

A tip of the *sombrero* goes to my friend Leah for her zesty South-of-the-Border recipe, which I've adapted for my own low fat needs.

If you do not like the (admittedly acquired) taste of cilantro, leave it out.

2 corn tortillas
2 teaspoons vegetable oil
6 scallions, white and tender greens, chopped
$^{1}/_{4}$ cup canned no-salt-added tomato sauce
4 cups Low Fat Chicken Stock (page 3) or canned low sodium broth
1 jalapeño pepper, seeded and finely chopped (wear gloves)
1 cup diced cooked turkey meat
$^{1}/_{4}$ teaspoon fresh lemon juice
Pinch cayenne pepper or to taste, optional
2 tablespoons chopped fresh coriander leaves (cilantro), optional

1. Cut tortillas into strips about $^{1}/_{4}$ inch wide and set aside.

2. Heat oil in a soup pot. Add scallions and cook, stirring, for 1 minute. Add all remaining ingredients, except tortilla strips and coriander, and bring to a simmer. Cover and cook for 10 minutes.

3. Add tortilla strips and cook for an additional 5

minutes. Ladle into heated bowls and serve garnished with coriander, if desired.

SERVES 4

Per serving: 135 calories; 12.0 grams protein; 9.5 grams carbohydrates; 5.5 grams fat; 29 milligrams cholesterol; 160 milligrams sodium (without salting).

DAY-AFTER-THANKSGIVING SOUP

Got lots of leftover turkey? Create a vegetable soup with some of the meat and any part of the bony carcass that's survived that midnight raid on the refrigerator. I also add baked sweet potatoes (peeled and diced) if there are any left over.

6 cups water
  Turkey bones or carcass
1 onion, chopped
2 stalks celery, chopped
1 carrot, cut into large dice
1 clove garlic, pressed
1 cup canned no-salt-added tomato sauce
¾ cup cooked or canned (drained and rinsed) kidney or
    pinto beans
1 cup chopped cooked turkey meat
1 tablespoon chopped fresh parsley
  Salt and freshly ground pepper to taste

1. Combine water and turkey bones or carcass in a large soup pot. Cover and bring to a simmer and cook for 1 hour. Strain, discarding bones.

2. Return soup to a simmer and add onion, celery, carrot, garlic, and tomato sauce. Cook for 15 to 20 minutes, covered, or until vegetables are tender.

3. Add beans, turkey, and parsley and cook until ingredients are heated through. Season to taste. Ladle into large heated bowls.

Serves 4

Per serving: 145 calories; 15.0 grams protein; 17.5 grams carbohydrates; 1.5 grams fat; 24 milligrams cholesterol; 65 milligrams sodium (without salting).

APPETIZERS
AND STARTERS

CHICKEN-FILLED
RED JACKET POTATOES

I find that everyone is enchanted with tiny new potatoes that are baked, and then stuffed with a spicy chicken mixture. This is a new version of the large twice-baked potatoes. Carefully scooping out the cooked potato from the small shells takes a bit of work, but the result is worth the effort.

12 small red jacket new potatoes, about 1½-inch
    diameter
1 teaspoon olive oil
¼ pound boneless and skinless chicken breasts, fat
    removed, ground or finely minced
1 teaspoon minced fresh parsley
⅛ teaspoon cayenne pepper, or to taste
½ cup low fat (2%) milk
Salt to taste

1. Preheat oven to 400° F.

2. Cut a very thin slice from one side of each potato to enable them to stand erect. Place potatoes on a shallow, nonstick baking pan and bake for about 45 minutes or until tender.

3. While potatoes bake, heat oil in a small nonstick skillet. Add chicken and sauté, stirring, for 5 to 8 minutes or until chicken is cooked through. Stir in parsley and cayenne, remove from heat and set aside.

4. When potatoes are tender, remove them from

oven and reduce oven temperature to 350° F. Let potatoes cool slightly.

5. Cut a ¼-inch slice from the top of each potato. Using a melon-ball cutter or a small spoon, carefully scoop out potato pulp, leaving shell intact. Transfer pulp to a medium saucepan.

6. Add milk to potato pulp and mash over low heat. Stir chicken mixture into potato and mix well to combine. Season to taste.

7. Spoon chicken-potato mixture into potato shells, mounding mixture carefully and smoothing top. Place filled potatoes on a baking sheet and return to oven for 5 to 10 minutes, or until hot.

SERVES 4

Per serving: 125 calories; 9.5 grams protein; 16.5 grams carbohydrates; 2.2 grams fat; 18 milligrams cholesterol; 40 milligrams sodium (without salting).

CHICKEN AND CORN
IN DIJON SAUCE

Because the corn is added to the skillet at the last minute, it retains its crunch and provides greater texture.

1/2 pound skinless and boneless chicken thighs, fat removed, cut into strips
2 teaspoons cider vinegar
1 teaspoon olive oil
1/2 cup Low Fat Chicken Stock (page 3) or canned low sodium broth
2 teaspoons Dijon mustard
3/4 cup fresh or frozen and thawed corn kernels
Salt and freshly ground pepper to taste
1 cup watercress sprigs

1. Combine chicken and vinegar in a bowl. Toss to mix and let marinate for 15 minutes.

2. Heat oil in a medium nonstick skillet. Add chicken and cook over medium-high heat, stirring, for 1 minute.

3. Add stock and mustard to skillet, reduce heat and let simmer, stirring frequently, for 5 to 8 minutes or until chicken is cooked through and sauce has thickened slightly.

4. Stir corn into skillet, season to taste and let simmer for 1 minute. Remove from heat.

5. Place watercress around the perimeter of a small

serving platter. Spoon chicken-corn mixture onto the center of platter and serve.

SERVES 4
Per serving: 120 calories; 12.5 grams protein; 8.5 grams carbohydrates; 3.9 grams fat; 49 milligrams cholesterol; 140 milligrams sodium (without salting).

GINGERED CHICKEN KEBABS

The Asian home cook has long known that marinades infuse meat and poultry with lots of flavor but add little or no fat. Here, cubes of skinless chicken breast are marinated in a classic combination of rich-tasting and fragrant ingredients that will produce a juicy and flavorful first course. This recipe is easily doubled for use as an entrée.

1 tablespoon grated, peeled ginger root
1 clove garlic, pressed
1 teaspoon sesame oil
   Juice of 1 large lime
1/2 pound skinless and boneless chicken breasts, fat
      removed, cut into 1-inch chunks
8 cherry tomatoes
1 medium green bell pepper, cut into 8 strips

1. Combine ginger, garlic, oil, and lime in a bowl. Mix thoroughly. Add chicken and toss to coat. Refrigerate and let marinate for 30 minutes, turning once or twice in the marinade.

2. Preheat oven to broil.

3. Dividing portions equally, thread chicken, tomatoes, and pepper strips onto four skewers. Place skewers on a broiling pan and spoon marinade over all.

4. Broil, turning skewers twice, for 8 to 10 minutes or until chicken is lightly browned and cooked through. Place skewers on platter and serve, or re-

move from skewers and serve on individual heated dishes.

SERVES 4
Per serving: 95 calories; 14.0 grams protein; 5.0 grams carbohydrates; 2.1 grams fat; 32 milligrams cholesterol; 45 milligrams sodium (without salting).

BRAISED ASIAN CHICKEN AND GREEN BEANS

Half the fun of cooking is experimenting with ingredients and flavors. I happen to favor the combination I've described below. But you might try shifting around and making up your own mix of vegetables with the chicken. For example, you might add sliced mushrooms along with sliced water chestnuts, or try it with Napa cabbage.

$1/2$ pound fresh green beans, preferably thin or french-cut

$1/2$ pound skinless and boneless chicken breasts, fat removed, cubed

$1/2$ cup Low Fat Chicken Stock (page 3) or canned low sodium broth

2 scallions, white and tender greens, minced

2 teaspoons rice wine vinegar

2 teaspoons low sodium soy sauce

$1/4$ teaspoon hot red pepper flakes or to taste

1. Remove strings from beans and break in half.

2. Combine beans, chicken, and stock in a wok or large skillet and bring to a boil. Reduce heat slightly and simmer, stirring, for 5 minutes.

3. Add scallions to skillet and continue cooking and stirring for an additional 3 to 5 minutes or until chicken is cooked through.

4. Add remaining ingredients and cook over high

heat, stirring, for 1 minute. Spoon onto a heated platter and serve.

SERVES 4

Per serving: 85 calories; 14.0 grams protein; 4.5 grams carbohydrates; 1.0 grams fat; 33 milligrams cholesterol; 150 milligrams sodium (without salting).

CHICKEN AND FENNEL VINAIGRETTE

The sparkling taste of fennel transforms plain poached chicken breasts into a very tasty low fat starter. Balsamic and white wine vinegar add a bright, fresh accent, while the scant touch of oil and chicken pan juices add richness to the mix.

$^1\!/_2$ pound skinless and boneless chicken breasts, fat removed
$^1\!/_4$ cup Low Fat Chicken Stock (page 3) or canned low sodium broth
1 small fennel bulb, thinly sliced
Salt and freshly ground pepper to taste
1 teaspoon olive oil
1 teaspoon white wine vinegar
1 teaspoon balsamic vinegar

1. Combine chicken and stock in a medium skillet. Cover and cook over low heat for about 10 minutes or until chicken is cooked through. Remove from heat, uncover, and let chicken and pan juices cool.

2. When chicken is cool enough to handle, remove from skillet using a slotted spoon and cut into $^1\!/_2$-inch cubes.

3. Transfer chicken to a salad bowl. Add fennel and salt and pepper to taste and toss to combine.

4. In a small bowl combine olive oil and vinegars. Mix well. Stir in pan juices and mix again. Pour over chicken and serve at room temperature or chilled.

SERVES 4

Per serving: 85 calories; 13.5 grams protein; 2.5 grams carbohydrates; 2.2 grams fat; 33 milligrams cholesterol; 60 milligrams sodium (without salting).

CHICKEN-STUFFED FRYING PEPPERS WITH PIQUANT TOMATO SAUCE

Frying peppers are a kind of long and thin, curved sweet pepper that can range in color from green to red. With the seeds removed, these peppers are excellent for frying or stuffing with a variety of fillings.

  1 teaspoon olive oil
  1/4 pound skinless and boneless chicken breasts, fat removed, ground or finely minced
  1/4 pound finely chopped mushrooms, wiped clean
  1 teaspoon chopped fresh parsley
    Salt and freshly ground pepper to taste
  4 Italian frying peppers
  1 cup canned no-salt-added tomato sauce
  1/4 teaspoon ground cumin or to taste
  1/4 teaspoon dried thyme
    Pinch cayenne pepper or to taste, optional

1. Preheat oven to 350° F.
2. Heat oil in a medium nonstick skillet. Add chicken and mushrooms and cook, stirring frequently, for 5 to 8 minutes or until chicken is cooked through. Stir in parsley, season to taste, and set aside.
3. Cut each pepper in half lengthwise. Remove seeds, and open each pepper half carefully. Using a small spoon, fill pepper halves with chicken mixture, smoothing chicken on top.

4. Combine tomato sauce with cumin and thyme. Mix well and spoon onto the bottom of a shallow baking pan. Place stuffed peppers on top of sauce, spooning a small amount of sauce over each pepper.

5. Bake for 20 to 25 minutes or until peppers are tender.

6. Place 2 pepper halves on individual heated dishes, spoon sauce from pan over peppers, and serve.

SERVES 4

Per serving: 75 calories; 8.0 grams protein; 7.0 grams carbohydrates; 1.9 grams fat; 16 milligrams cholesterol; 35 milligrams sodium (without salting).

TURKEY TORTILLAS
WITH HOT SALSA

The rap against Mexican food is that it's heavy with fat and therefore unsuitable for today's lighter style of eating. Well, it isn't necessarily so, as my recipe for Turkey Tortillas illustrates.

6 plum tomatoes, peeled, seeded, and finely chopped
4 scallions, white and tender greens, minced
2 teaspoons hot pepper sauce
1 teaspoon olive oil
  Olive oil cooking spray
1/2 pound ground lean turkey
  Salt and freshly ground pepper to taste
4 corn tortillas
1 small green bell pepper, sliced into thin rings

1. Preheat oven to 325° F.
2. To make salsa, combine tomatoes, scallion, hot pepper sauce, and oil in a small bowl. Mix well and set aside.
3. Wrap tortillas in foil and place in oven to warm.
4. Heat cooking spray in a medium nonstick skillet. Add turkey and cook, stirring frequently, for 8 to 10 minutes or until turkey is cooked through. Season to taste.
5. Remove tortillas from oven. Spoon one-quarter of the turkey onto a tortilla. Add 1 teaspoon of salsa and roll. Repeat with remaining tortillas.
6. Place tortillas on individual serving dishes and

garnish with remaining salsa and pepper rings. Serve immediately.

SERVES 4
Per serving: 185 calories; 12.0 grams protein; 18.0 grams carbohydrates; 6.8 grams fat; 44 milligrams cholesterol; 110 milligrams sodium (without salting).

SMOKED TURKEY
AND EGGPLANT ROLL-UPS

The best eggplant for this dish are the small Italian or Asian eggplant. These are not bitter, have the tiniest of seeds, and their mild flavor is a fine counterpoint to the smoky flavor of the turkey.

Olive oil cooking spray
2 small Italian or Asian eggplant (about 8 ounces total), each cut lengthwise into 4 slices
Salt and freshly ground pepper to taste
8 thin slices smoked turkey breast (about 1/4 pound total)
12 cherry tomatoes

1. Preheat oven to 350° F.
2. Coat a large, shallow baking pan with cooking spray. Place eggplant slices in pan in a single layer and bake for about 15 minutes or until tender. Season eggplant to taste and set aside until cool enough to handle.
3. Place a slice of turkey on each eggplant slice and roll, securing with a toothpick.
4. Place roll-ups on a serving platter, garnish with cherry tomatoes, and serve.

SERVES 4
Per serving: 75 calories; 7.5 grams protein; 8.5 grams carbohydrates; 1.3 grams fat; 18 milligrams cholesterol; 300 milligrams sodium (without salting).

TURKEY BALLS
IN TOMATO-ONION CONFIT

"Confit" is an ancient method of preserving meat—usually goose or duck—whereby cooked meat is packed into a crock or pot and covered with its own cooking fat. In my low fat version, lightly sautéed vegetables—*not* turkey fat—serve as the "confit"; that is, they seal in the flavor of a delightful ground turkey mixture that is shaped into tiny balls. I must confess, I often mash the whole lot together and spread it on good, crusty French or Italian bread and have it for lunch!

1 teaspoon olive oil
6 plum tomatoes, chopped
2 onions, diced
1/4 teaspoon ground cumin or to taste
1/4 teaspoon hot paprika or to taste
1 tablespoon chopped fresh basil or 2 teaspoons dried
  Salt to taste
1/2 pound ground lean turkey
  Egg substitute equal to 1 egg
1 slice thin-sliced white bread softened in water

1. Heat oil in a medium nonstick saucepan. Add tomatoes, onion, cumin, and paprika. Cover and cook over very low heat, stirring occasionally, until vegetables are thoroughly cooked and combined. Stir in basil and remove from heat. Taste and add salt and correct seasoning, if desired. Set aside.

2. Combine turkey, egg substitute, and bread in a medium bowl. Mash until mixture is thoroughly blended, then shape into tiny balls.

3. Add turkey balls to tomato-onion mixture in saucepan and return to heat. Cook, stirring frequently, over low heat for 8 to 10 minutes or until turkey is cooked through. Transfer turkey and confit to a shallow bowl or individual dishes and serve.

SERVES 4

Per serving: 175 calories; 13.5 grams protein; 15.5 grams carbohydrates; 6.5 grams fat; 44 milligrams cholesterol; 120 milligrams sodium (without salting).

WONDERFUL HASH

I've named this dish, which is made with leftover chicken or turkey, Wonderful Hash because that's the comment I hear most often when I serve it to guests. Yes, guests! Hash is no longer a dish that can be served only to understanding family members. I like to serve this hash as an interesting starter, but the recipe may also be doubled and served as a main course.

1 medium potato, baked
1/4 cup low fat (2%) milk
1 small onion, minced
1 small green bell pepper, diced
1 cup leftover shredded cooked chicken or turkey
1 tablespoon ketchup
Salt and freshly ground pepper to taste
Vegetable oil cooking spray

1. Preheat oven to 400° F.

2. Scoop baked potato pulp from shell into a small bowl. Add milk, onion, green bell pepper and mix well. Stir in chicken or turkey and ketchup. Mix again and season to taste.

3. Spoon hash mixture into a small, shallow oven-proof pan lightly coated with cooking spray. Bake for about 10 minutes or until top is lightly browned.

4. Using a pie cutter, slice hash into 4 wedges, and serve.

Per serving: 105 calories; 11.0 grams protein; 9.5 grams carbohydrates; 2.7 grams fat; 27 milligrams cholesterol; 75 milligrams sodium (without salting).

TURKEY SATAY
WITH PEANUT SAUCE

Thai food has become increasingly popular in recent years and lemongrass is one of the most important flavorings in Thai cooking. Lemongrass has long, thin gray-green leaves and a scallionlike base, and is available dried and fresh in specialty produce markets. It has a divinely sour-lemon taste and fragrance. In a pinch, substitute lemon peel.

This recipe may be prepared with small metal skewers; however, presoaked-soaked bamboo makes for easy handling and more even, and authentic, cooking.

$^1/_2$ pound turkey breast cutlets

1 clove garlic, quartered

1 piece peeled ginger, about $1^1/_2$ inches long, cut in pieces

$^1/_4$ teaspoon ground turmeric

2 stalks lemongrass, optional

2 teaspoons low sodium soy sauce

$^1/_4$ cup orange juice

2 teaspoons brown sugar

8 bamboo skewers, soaked in cold water for 30 minutes

PEANUT SAUCE

2 tablespoons salt-free creamy peanut butter

1 clove garlic

$^1/_4$ cup fresh lime juice

$^1/_2$ teaspoon sesame oil

¹/₂ teaspoon white wine vinegar
¹/₄ cup pineapple juice

1. Pound turkey cutlets to ¹/₄-inch thickness between sheets of plastic wrap. Cut turkey into slices approximately ¹/₂ inches wide by 3 inches long. Place in a shallow bowl.

2. Combine garlic, ginger, turmeric, lemongrass, soy sauce, orange juice, and sugar in a food processor and process until mixture forms into a paste. Spoon mixture onto turkey and toss. Cover bowl and set aside to marinate for about 30 minutes.

3. While meat marinates, prepare Peanut Sauce by combining all sauce ingredients in a food processor. Process until thoroughly blended. Spoon sauce into a small serving bowl and set aside.

4. Preheat broiler.

5. Thread meat onto bamboo skewers and place on a broiler pan or a baking sheet. Broil, turning once, for 5 to 7 minutes or until meat is cooked through.

6. Place skewers on a serving platter or individual dishes and offer sauce on the side.

SERVES 4

Per serving: 150 calories; 16.5 grams protein; 9.5 grams carbohydrates; 5.3 grams fat; 36 milligrams cholesterol; 130 milligrams sodium (without salting).

TURKEY AND BROWN RICE QUICHE

I constantly find myself entangled in good cooking challenges, where I have to wrestle with high fat, high calorie favorites and try to turn them into healthful, good-tasting dishes my guests and I will really love.

Quiches present such a challenge because they are traditionally made with a pastry shell filled with a savory custard consisting of eggs, cream, seasonings, and various other ingredients. My recipe, which omits the pastry, cream, and egg yolks, is absolutely delicious—and it keeps the total fat down to nutritionally sound levels, too!

Vegetable oil cooking spray
2 cups cooked brown rice, at room temperature
1 1/2 cups chopped cooked turkey
1 tomato, diced
4 scallions, white and tender greens, chopped
1 small green bell pepper, diced
1 tablespoon chopped fresh parsley
1/4 teaspoon cayenne pepper or to taste
Salt to taste
3/4 cup shredded low fat cheddar cheese (about 3 ounces)
1/2 cup low fat (1%) milk
Egg substitute equal to 4 eggs

1. Preheat oven to 350° F. Coat a 9- × 13-inch pan or ovenproof casserole with cooking spray and set aside.

2. In a large mixing bowl, combine all ingredients, except milk and egg substitute. Toss to blend ingredients. Add milk and egg substitute and stir until all ingredients are thoroughly blended.

3. Spoon rice-turkey mixture into prepared pan or casserole and bake for about 30 minutes or until a knife inserted in center comes out clean.

4. Let stand 2 minutes before serving.

SERVES 4

Per serving: 305 calories; 30.0 grams protein; 28.5 grams carbohydrates; 7.5 grams fat; 53 milligrams cholesterol; 210 milligrams sodium (without salting).

SALADS AND LIGHT MEALS

CHICKEN SALAD WITH CREAMY TARRAGON DRESSING

Tarragon is one of the "can't-do-without" herbs on my spice rack. Known for its distinctive aroma and aniselike flavor, it's an integral ingredient in many herbal combinations, such as *fines herbes,* as well as sauces, such as béarnaise. Since its assertiveness can easily dominate other flavors, a light hand is recommended.

  1/3 cup low fat sour cream
  1/3 cup low fat plain yogurt
  2 teaspoons fresh lemon juice
  3/4 teaspoon dried tarragon or to taste
  2 tablespoons chopped fresh parsley
    Salt and freshly ground pepper to taste
  2 cups cubed cooked chicken breast
  4 scallions, white and tender greens, minced
  2 stalks celery, finely chopped
  1 head Bibb lettuce, rinsed, dried, and separated into leaves
  1 small cucumber, peeled and sliced into thin rings

1. Combine sour cream, yogurt, lemon juice, tarragon, parsley, and salt and pepper in a small bowl and whisk until ingredients are thoroughly and smoothly blended.

2. Place chicken in a medium bowl with scallions and celery. Spoon on dressing and toss to coat all ingredients. Taste and adjust seasoning if necessary.

3. Arrange lettuce leaves on individual serving plates, top with spoonfuls of chicken salad mixture, surround with cucumber slices, and serve.

SERVES 4
Per serving: 160 calories; 22.0 grams protein; 5.5 grams carbohydrates; 5.4 grams fat; 60 milligrams cholesterol; 85 milligrams sodium (without salting).

CHICKEN SALAD WITH SWEET-AND-SOUR PEARL ONIONS

Baking intensifies the flavor of the onions and adds richness to this sophisticated salad combination.

Olive oil cooking spray
12 small pearl onions, peeled
1 teaspoon sugar
1 tablespoon red wine vinegar
3/4 pound skinless and boneless chicken breasts, fat removed
1/2 cup Low Fat Chicken Stock (page 3) or canned low sodium broth
1/2 teaspoon dried rosemary
1 cup shredded romaine lettuce
Salt and freshly ground pepper to taste

1. Preheat oven to 350° F.

2. Coat a small, shallow baking pan with cooking spray. Cut a cross in the root end of each onion and place in baking pan. Combine sugar and vinegar in a bowl, mix well, spoon over onions and toss. Bake in oven for about 30 minutes or until onions are tender.

3. While onions bake, combine chicken, stock, and rosemary in a small skillet. Cover and simmer over medium heat for about 10 minutes or until chicken is tender. Using a slotted spoon, remove chicken from skillet and set aside to cool. Add juices from skillet to onions as they bake.

4. When onions are tender remove from oven and spoon with contents of baking pan into a medium bowl. Allow to cool slightly.

5. When chicken has cooled, cut into small cubes. Add cubed chicken to onions in bowl, season to taste with salt and pepper, and toss gently.

6. Create a bed of romaine lettuce on a serving platter. Top with chicken-onion combination. Serve at room temperature.

SERVES 4

Per serving: 115 calories; 20.5 grams protein; 4.0 grams carbohydrates; 2.0 grams fat; 49 milligrams cholesterol; 135 milligrams sodium (without salting).

LEMON-MARINATED CHICKEN WITH RADICCHIO AND ENDIVE

This exquisite salad beautifully balances flavors and tastes so that you won't miss the dimension of fat. There's lemon in the chicken for a sour taste; for sweetness, a touch of honey in the dressing, and I've chosen radicchio and endive specifically for their crunch and pleasantly bitter bite.

1/2 pound skinless and boneless chicken breast, fat removed
Juice of 1 large lemon
1/2 teaspoon freshly ground pepper
Salt to taste
3 teaspoons olive oil
1 teaspoon balsamic vinegar
1/2 teaspoon honey
1 small head radicchio, torn into small pieces
1 Belgian endive, separated into leaves

1. Cut chicken into thin slices and place in a shallow dish. Sprinkle with lemon juice and season with pepper. Toss to combine and allow chicken to marinate at room temperature for 15 minutes. Turn chicken in marinade once or twice.

2. Heat 1 teaspoon oil in a medium nonstick skillet. Remove chicken from marinade and pat dry. Sauté chicken over medium-high heat, turning to brown lightly on all sides, until chicken is done. Remove

chicken from skillet with a slotted spoon and set aside to cool.

3. Combine remaining 2 teaspoons oil with vinegar and honey in a small bowl. Mix well. Spoon dressing over radicchio and toss.

4. Arrange radicchio in center of a serving platter and top with chicken slices. Place endive leaves around perimeter of platter and serve.

SERVES 4

Per serving: 120 calories; 15.0 grams protein; 6.0 grams carbohydrates; 4.5 grams fat; 32 milligrams cholesterol; 20 milligrams sodium (without salting).

CHICKEN TOSS WITH SPINACH PASTA AND DRIED TOMATOES

Here's a dish that's as colorful as it is delicious. The combination of colors—the creamy whiteness of chicken, emerald green pasta, and Burgundy-red tomatoes—makes for a most attractive salad.

  Vegetable oil cooking spray
2 chicken thighs (about ¹/₂ pound)
  Salt and freshly ground pepper to taste
¹/₄ pound spinach pasta (twists, farfalle, or shells)
2 ounces no-salt-added dried tomatoes
2 teaspoons olive oil
1 teaspoon cider vinegar

1. Preheat oven to 350° F.
2. Coat a shallow baking pan with cooking spray. Place chicken in pan, season to taste, and cover with foil. Bake for about 30 minutes or until chicken is cooked through. Remove chicken from oven and allow to cool until it can be easily handled.
3. While chicken bakes, cook pasta in a large pot of boiling water until just done. Drain and transfer to a medium bowl. Allow pasta to cool.
4. Soften dried tomatoes in boiling water to cover for 5 minutes. Drain and chop finely.
5. Combine oil and vinegar and mix well. Stir in chopped dried tomatoes. Spoon oil-vinegar combination over pasta, mix thoroughly and set aside.
6. When chicken has cooled, remove skin and cut

meat from bone. Cut chicken meat into small cubes and discard skin and bones.

7. Add chicken to pasta and toss to combine. Season to taste and transfer to a serving platter. Serve at room temperature.

SERVES 4
Per serving: 215 calories; 12.0 grams protein; 31.0 grams carbohydrates; 5.0 grams fat; 29 milligrams cholesterol; 50 milligrams sodium (without salting).

ASIAN CHICKEN SALAD WITH ANGEL HAIR PASTA

Five-spice powder is used extensively in Chinese cooking. It is a pungent mixture of five ground spices—consisting of equal parts of cinnamon, cloves, fennel seed, star anise, and Szechuan peppercorns—and it is available in jars in many supermarkets and Asian food stores. I have found it indispensable in my low fat cooking scheme.

    1 whole chicken breast (about 1 pound)
      Herb bouquet: 4 sprigs fresh parsley, bay leaf, and 4
        sprigs dill, tied together
    6 ounces angel hair pasta or cappellini
    2 teaspoons sesame oil
    2 teaspoons low sodium soy sauce
  1/4 teaspoon hot pepper sauce
      Pinch Chinese 5-spice powder or to taste
    4 scallions, with tops, finely chopped
    1 tablespoon rice wine vinegar
  1/2 small head iceberg lettuce, shredded

1. Place chicken in a medium saucepan. Add water to cover by 2 inches and add herb bouquet. Cover, bring to a simmer and cook for 20 minutes or until tender. Remove chicken from liquid and let stand until cool enough to handle.

2. Meanwhile, cook pasta in a large pot of boiling water until al dente. Drain, place in a medium bowl,

and toss with 1 teaspoon sesame oil. Set aside to cool slightly.

3. When chicken is cooled, remove and discard skin and bones. Cut chicken meat into strips.

4. Combine remaining teaspoon sesame oil with soy sauce, hot pepper sauce, and 5-spice powder in a medium bowl. Mix well and toss with chicken.

5. Add scallions and rice wine vinegar to pasta in bowl and mix until combined.

6. Place a bed of shredded lettuce on a serving platter. Top with pasta and spoon chicken over pasta. Serve at room temperature.

SERVES 4

Per serving: 250 calories; 19.5 grams protein; 33.0 grams carbohydrates; 4.0 grams fat; 32 milligrams cholesterol; 155 milligrams sodium (without salting).

ROMAN-STYLE CHICKEN AND RICE SALAD

When I was visiting Italy some years ago, I sampled—no, "scarfed"—a dish that was very similar to the one I've adapted here. The red bell pepper adds color and crunch, and I find this salad to be a wonderful part of any buffet table.

  1 whole chicken breast (about 1 pound)
    Salt and freshly ground pepper to taste
  2 tablespoons red wine vinegar
  1 tablespoon olive oil
  1 teaspoon Dijon mustard
2 1/2 cups cooked rice, at room temperature
  1 red bell pepper, trimmed, seeded, and diced
  3 slices sweet pickle chips, diced

1. Place chicken in a medium saucepan. Add water to cover by 2 inches and season to taste with salt and pepper. Bring to a simmer, cover, and cook for about 15 minutes or until chicken is cooked through. Remove chicken from liquid and set aside to cool until it can be easily handled.

2. Combine vinegar, oil, and mustard in a small bowl, and mix well. Spoon over rice in a large bowl and toss to combine ingredients.

3. When chicken is cool, remove skin and cut meat off bones. Cut chicken meat into a fine dice, and discard skin and bones.

4. Add diced chicken, bell pepper, and pickle to rice

and mix all ingredients thoroughly. Serve at room temperature.

SERVES 4

Per serving: 270 calories; 17.0 grams protein; 39.0 grams carbohydrates; 4.7 grams fat; 32 milligrams cholesterol; 120 milligrams sodium (without salting).

INDIAN-SPICED CHICKEN SALAD WITH BASMATI RICE

Basmati rice from India has a flavor and aroma that brings a lot more to the party than the usual long-grain rice. Basmati comes directly from India, but there's also an American version called texmati. You may use either for this recipe and follow cooking direction on the package. I've discovered that directions may vary according to the brand of rice I buy.

Serve either at room temperature or chilled.

½ chicken breast (about ½ pound)
*   Salt and freshly ground pepper to taste*
1 cup low fat plain yogurt
1 clove garlic, pressed
¼ teaspoon ground turmeric
¼ teaspoon ground cumin
1 small Kirby cucumber, diced
1 cup basmati rice, cooked and cooled slightly
1 tablespoon chopped fresh cilantro or basil

1. Preheat broiler.

2. Season chicken and place on a broiling pan, skin side up. Broil about 6 to 8 minutes on each side, or until chicken is done. Set aside until cool enough to handle.

3. While chicken cools, combine yogurt, garlic, turmeric, cumin, and cucumber in a small bowl. Mix until thoroughly combined.

4. When chicken is cool, remove and discard skin

and bones. Cut meat into cubes in a small bowl. Combine cubed chicken with one-half of yogurt mixture and mix well.

5. Combine rice with remaining yogurt mixture in a small bowl and mix well.

6. Spoon rice onto a serving platter and top with chicken mixture. Garnish with cilantro or basil and serve.

SERVES 4

Per serving: 130 calories; 11.5 grams protein; 17.5 grams carbohydrates; 1.3 grams fat; 20 milligrams cholesterol; 65 milligrams sodium (without salting).

SAVORY CHICKEN-STUFFED ONIONS

Vidalia onions, those exceptionally sweet onions, are best for this dish, but if they're not available substitute either Bermuda or Spanish onions.

4 large onions, preferably Vidalia
1/4 cup Low Fat Chicken Stock (page 3) or canned low sodium broth
Salt and freshly ground pepper to taste
Pinch cayenne pepper or to taste
1/2 pound skinless and boneless chicken breasts, fat removed
1/2 cup cooked brown rice
1/4 teaspoon ground cumin
1/4 cup bread crumbs

1. Peel onions without cutting off root ends. Place onions in boiling water and cook for 10 minutes. Remove onions from water and allow to cool.

2. Combine stock, salt, pepper, cayenne, and chicken in a medium skillet. Cover and cook over medium heat for 5 to 8 minutes or until chicken is tender and cooked through. Remove chicken from skillet and allow to cool.

3. Preheat oven to 350° F.

4. Cut a slice off from top of each onion. Scoop out the centers of each onion to form a hollow, being careful not to cut through bottom. Finely chop scooped-out part. Transfer to a medium bowl.

5. Cut chicken meat into small cubes and add to chopped onion.

6. Add rice and cumin to chicken-onion mixture, and stir until combined.

7. Using a small spoon stuff each onion with chicken-rice mixture. Sprinkle tops with bread crumbs.

8. Place onions in a shallow baking pan and add water just to cover bottom of the pan. Bake for 20 to 30 minutes or until crumbs have browned and all ingredients are heated through. Serve warm or at room temperature.

SERVES 4

Per serving: 175 calories; 16.5 grams protein; 25.0 grams carbohydrates; 1.3 grams fat; 33 milligrams cholesterol; 70 milligrams sodium (without salting).

GRILLED CHICKEN SOUVLAKI IN PITA

This Greek specialty is particularly appealing to kids and to those of us who like to think (and eat) young. Normally the dish is made with marinated chunks of lamb that are skewered and grilled, but the idea of using chicken in its stead makes a lot of heart-healthy sense.

3/4 pound skinless and boneless chicken breasts, fat
   removed, cut into 2-inch pieces
2 teaspoons red wine vinegar
2 teaspoons olive oil
2 cloves garlic, pressed
1/2 teaspoon each: dried oregano, thyme, and rosemary
   Salt and freshly ground pepper to taste
1 cup low fat plain yogurt
4 large pitas
2 just-ripe plum tomatoes, coarsely chopped
2 cups shredded lettuce
1 small onion, thinly sliced

1. Combine vinegar, oil, 1 clove garlic, herbs, and salt and pepper in a small bowl. Mix well.

2. Place chicken in a shallow bowl. Add vinegar mixture and turn chicken to coat all sides. Cover and refrigerate for 1 hour, turning chicken once.

3. Prepare grill or preheat broiler.

4. Combine yogurt with remaining garlic and set aside.

5. Thread chicken onto metal skewers and grill or broil 4 to 5 inches from heat for about 5 minutes on each side or until cooked through, brushing with remaining marinade.

6. While chicken cooks, cut off a small piece from each pita to make an opening and heat pitas briefly.

7. Divide chicken pieces and remaining ingredients evenly among pitas. Add a large dollop of yogurt mixture to each and serve.

SERVES 4

Per serving: 305 calories; 28.0 grams protein; 38.5 grams carbohydrates; 5.2 grams fat; 51 milligrams cholesterol; 500 milligrams sodium (without salting).

SMOKED TURKEY
AND WHITE BEAN SALAD

This tasty salad can be put together in a jiffy if you use canned beans—but if you do, be sure to rinse and drain the beans well.

  1 cup cooked or canned white beans
    Salt and freshly ground pepper to taste
  2 teaspoons olive oil
  2 teaspoons red wine vinegar
  1 teaspoon balsamic vinegar
  1 medium red onion, thinly sliced and separated into
      rings
  ³/₄ pound smoked breast of turkey, sliced and cut into
      thin strips
  2 cups shredded chicory or lettuce

1. Place beans in a medium bowl and season with salt and pepper.

2. In a separate bowl, combine oil and vinegars. Mix thoroughly and spoon over beans.

3. In another bowl, combine onion and turkey and toss to mix.

4. Place shredded chicory or lettuce on a serving platter. Spoon beans onto center of the platter. Top beans with onion-turkey mixture and serve.

SERVES 4
Per serving: 195 calories; 22.0 grams protein; 17.5 grams carbohydrates; 4.0 grams fat; 39.0 milligrams cholesterol; 750 milligrams sodium (without salting).

TURKEY AND BELL PEPPER SALAD IN ZUCCHINI BOATS

This is best served at room temperature, but it can be made in advance and refrigerated for a chilled summer treat.

2 medium zucchini, about 6 inches long
6 plum tomatoes, finely chopped
1 small onion, minced
$1/4$ teaspoon dried oregano
$1/2$ teaspoon hot pepper sauce
2 teaspoons olive oil
$3/4$ pound turkey breast cutlets
Salt and freshly ground pepper to taste
1 small red or yellow bell pepper, trimmed, seeded, and diced

1. Place zucchini in a medium pot of boiling water to cover and cook until just tender (zucchini should retain shape). Remove from water and set aside to cool.

3. Combine tomatoes, onion, oregano, and hot pepper sauce in a small bowl. Mix well and set aside.

4. Heat oil in a large nonstick skillet. Place turkey in skillet in one layer and season with salt and pepper. Cook over medium-low heat, turning from side to side, for about 15 minutes or until lightly brown and cooked through. Remove from skillet and set aside to cool.

5. Cut each zucchini in half lengthwise. Scoop out

seeds and some pulp, being careful to keep shell intact. Pat zucchini shells dry with paper towels and set aside.

6. Cut turkey into a fine dice and combine with diced bell pepper in a medium bowl. Add tomato sauce mixture to turkey and stir until combined.

7. Spoon turkey mixture into and around zucchini boats and serve.

SERVES 4

Per serving: 170 calories; 23.5 grams protein; 12.0 grams carbohydrates; 3.5 grams fat; 54 milligrams cholesterol; 70 milligrams sodium (without salting).

TURKEY WALDORF SALAD

The original version of this salad, which is said to have been created at New York's Waldorf-Astoria Hotel many moons ago, contained only apples, celery, and mayonnaise. It was much later that walnuts became identified with the dish. I've taken it a couple of steps further and included turkey and grapes—plus I've streamlined the dressing ingredients so that we have a kind of Waldorf Spa Salad. Serve it chilled or at room temperature.

   1 large McIntosh apple
   2 teaspoons fresh lemon juice
   ³/₄ pound skinless and boneless turkey breast, cooked and
       cut into ¹/₂-inch cubes
   2 stalks celery, diced
   1 cup seedless white or red grapes
   2 tablespoons chopped walnuts
   ¹/₂ cup low fat plain yogurt
   ¹/₃ cup low fat mayonnaise
   ¹/₂ teaspoon celery seeds
       Salt and freshly ground pepper to taste
   4 cups shredded romaine lettuce leaves

1. Cut apple in half, core, and cut into 1-inch cubes. Place apple in a large mixing bowl and toss with lemon juice. Add turkey, celery, grapes, and walnuts.

2. In a separate bowl, combine yogurt, mayonnaise, celery seeds, and salt and pepper. Whisk until ingredients are smoothly and thoroughly blended.

3. Spoon yogurt mixture onto apple-turkey mixture in bowl and toss until ingredients are coated with dressing.

4. Arrange lettuce leaves on 4 serving plates, top with equal amounts of turkey salad, and serve.

SERVES 4

Per serving: 275 calories; 29.5 grams protein; 15.5 grams carbohydrates; 10.5 grams fat; 80 milligrams cholesterol; 245 milligrams sodium (without salting).

CHILLED TURKEY, BROCCOLI, AND FENNEL SALAD

I've tried all kinds of reduced-fat dressings, from store-bought to homemade, and I believe my garlicky ranch-style dressing below is one of the best of its kind.

2 cups broccoli florets
³/₄ pound turkey breast cutlets, cooked and cubed
1 small fennel bulb, thinly sliced
6 scallions, white and tender greens, chopped
2 cloves garlic, quartered
2 teaspoons olive oil
¹/₂ cup low fat (2%) cottage cheese
2 tablespoons low fat sour cream
2 tablespoons skim milk, approximately
¹/₄ cup chopped fresh parsley
  Salt and freshly ground pepper to taste
3 cups cut romaine or Boston lettuce leaves

1. In a medium saucepan, cook broccoli in boiling water to cover for about 5 minutes or until just fork-tender. Drain, rinse with cold water, then drain again.

2. Combine broccoli with turkey, fennel, and scallions in a large mixing bowl and toss lightly. Cover and refrigerate for at least 1 hour to chill.

3. In a food processor, combine garlic and oil and process until garlic is coarsely pureed. Add all remaining ingredients, except lettuce, and process until smoothly pureed; add additional skim milk if dressing

is too thick. Cover and refrigerate until turkey mixture is chilled.

4. Spoon dressing onto broccoli-turkey mixture and toss to blend.

5. Arrange lettuce on a platter or individual plates, top with turkey-broccoli salad, and serve.

SERVES 4
Per serving: 220 calories; 33.0 grams protein; 10.5 grams carbohydrates; 5.0 grams fat; 78 milligrams cholesterol; 225 milligrams sodium (without salting).

TANGY TURKEY BURGERS ON ENGLISH MUFFINS

Because turkey is so lean, it needs moisturizing ingredients to replace the missing fat. The blend of vegetables, seasonings, and binders in my recipe produce a juicy burger with lots of zing and little fat. It also works well when shaped into a meat loaf.

    1 pound ground turkey
    1/2 cup grated carrot
    1 small onion, finely minced
    1 clove garlic, pressed
      Egg substitute equal to 1 egg
    2 teaspoons Dijon mustard
    1 tablespoon Worcestershire sauce
      Salt and freshly ground pepper to taste
    1/2 tablespoon vegetable oil
    4 English muffins
    4 tablespoons low sodium ketchup
    1/4 teaspoon hot pepper sauce or to taste, optional
      Shredded lettuce leaves
    4 thin slices red onion

1. In a large mixing bowl, combine turkey, carrot, onion, and garlic. Mix until well blended. Add egg substitute, mustard, Worcestershire sauce, and salt and pepper to taste. Mix again to blend all ingredients. Form into 4 patties.

2. Heat oil in a large nonstick skillet. Add turkey

patties and cook over medium heat for 5 to 7 minutes on each side or until browned and cooked through.

3. About 2 to 3 minutes before burgers are done, split muffins and toast lightly. Spread both sides of muffins with ketchup mixed with hot pepper sauce if desired.

4. Arrange lettuce on one-half of each muffin. Top lettuce with a burger and an onion slice, and serve immediately.

SERVES 4

Per serving: 360 calories; 26.5 grams protein; 34.5 grams carbohydrates; 12.5 grams fat; 88 milligrams cholesterol; 465 milligrams sodium (without salting).

THE MAIN DISH:
BAKED AND
ROASTED

ROASTED CHICKEN BREAST WITH ELEPHANT GARLIC SAUCE

Elephant garlic is the mammoth garlic bulb that's about the size of a small orange. This huge garlic has a milder taste than its smaller brother, and can be sliced and added to dishes without fear of overpowering the main ingredient.

If elephant garlic is not available prepare this recipe with regular garlic, reducing the number of cloves by half. Remember that garlic is considerably tamed as it cooks.

  2 whole small chicken breasts (about 12 ounces each),
      skin and fat removed, split
      Salt and freshly ground pepper to taste
      Paprika to taste
  6 cloves elephant garlic or 3 cloves regular garlic,
      unpeeled
1½ cups Low Fat Chicken Stock (page 3) or canned low
      sodium broth
  ¼ cup dry white wine

1. Preheat oven to 375° F.

2. Season chicken on all sides with salt and pepper. Sprinkle top side of chicken with paprika. Place chicken, paprika side up, in a roasting pan and strew garlic cloves around chicken. Add stock or broth.

3. Roast, covered, for 15 minutes. Remove cover and baste. Continue roasting, uncovered, for an additional 30 to 40 minutes or until chicken is browned

and cooked through. Remove chicken to a serving platter and keep warm.

4. Transfer pan juices to a small saucepan. Using a slotted spoon, remove garlic cloves.

5. Pop the garlic cloves out of their skins by gently squeezing between the fingers.

6. Add garlic cloves and wine to saucepan. Bring to a simmer, and reduce by one-third, stirring and pressing garlic cloves with the back of a large spoon. Pour garlic sauce over chicken. Serve hot.

SERVES 4

Per serving: 105 calories; 20.0 grams protein; 2.5 grams carbohydrates; 1.8 grams fat; 50 milligrams cholesterol; 80 milligrams sodium (without salting).

BRANDIED ROAST CHICKEN WITH CREAMED MUSHROOMS AND PEAS

This elegant dish makes a beautiful presentation that would be suitable for any "company" meal. The cream in the sauce is provided by just two tablespoons of low fat sour cream, so don't be put off.

1 3-pound chicken, skin and fat removed, cut into 8 pieces
1/2 cup dry white wine
1/2 cup brandy
1/2 teaspoon dried thyme
1/2 teaspoon dried tarragon
Salt and freshly ground pepper to taste
Vegetable oil cooking spray
3/4 cup Low Fat Chicken Stock (page 3) or canned low sodium broth
2 shallots, minced
1/2 pound small mushrooms, wiped clean and thinly sliced
1/2 cup fresh or frozen green peas
1 tablespoon fine flour
2 tablespoons low fat sour cream

1. Place chicken in a shallow pan. Combine wine, brandy, thyme, and tarragon in a small bowl and pour over chicken, turning to coat all sides. Cover and refrigerate for 4 hours, turning chicken pieces every 30 minutes.

2. Preheat oven to 375° F.

3. Remove chicken from marinade and season with salt and pepper. Place chicken pieces in a roasting pan coated with cooking spray and roast, basting occasionally with marinade, for 45 minutes to 1 hour or until chicken is tender and cooked through.

4. While chicken roasts, combine ¹/₂ cup stock, shallots, and mushrooms in a medium saucepan and cook over medium-low heat, stirring occasionally, for 10 minutes. Add peas and cook an additional 3 to 5 minutes or until peas and mushrooms are tender. Remove from heat and set aside.

5. When chicken is cooked, remove from oven. Transfer chicken to a platter and keep warm. Place roasting pan with its contents over low heat. Deglaze with remaining stock, stirring over high heat. Sprinkle with flour and stir until dissolved. Add mushrooms and contents of saucepan to roasting pan, and stir until ingredients are combined and slightly thickened. Remove from heat and stir in sour cream.

6. Spoon mushrooms and sauce over and around chicken pieces on platter and serve immediately.

SERVES 4

Per serving: 265 calories; 38.0 grams protein; 11.5 grams carbohydrates; 7.1 grams fat; 116 milligrams cholesterol; 150 milligrams sodium (without salting).

BAKED CHICKEN TAHITIAN

The fresh pineapple cubes make a taste difference in this Island-inspired recipe, but if you absolutely must, canned and drained pineapple may be substituted.

    1 large tomato, peeled, seeded, and chopped
    1 medium onion, chopped
    1 teaspoon olive oil
1½ cups Low Fat Chicken Stock (page 3) or canned low
        sodium broth
    1 3-pound chicken, skin and fat removed, quartered
    2 bananas, peeled and cut lengthwise in half
    1 cup fresh pineapple cubes
  ¼ cup dry sherry

1. Preheat oven to 400° F.
2. Combine tomato, onion, and oil in a medium saucepan. Cook over low heat, stirring frequently, for about 5 minutes or until ingredients are combined and liquid has been reduced. Add 1 cup of the stock, a quarter of a cup at a time, and continue cooking, uncovered, over low heat until ingredients are blended and reduced by a third.
3. Place chicken pieces in a shallow baking pan and add remainder of stock. Bake, basting every 15 minutes, for about 45 minutes or until chicken is tender and cooked through. Add bananas during last 5 minutes.

4. Add pineapple to reduced tomato-stock mixture in saucepan and cook for 2 minutes.

5. Remove chicken from baking pan and place on a platter. Place banana pieces beside chicken and keep warm.

6. Add sherry to baking pan and combine with pan juices. Mix well and add to pineapple-tomato combination in saucepan. Heat to a simmer, pour over chicken and bananas, and serve hot.

SERVES 4

Per serving: 315 calories; 37.0 grams protein; 25.5 grams carbohydrates; 7.5 grams fat; 117 milligrams cholesterol; 160 milligrams sodium (without salting).

CHICKEN BAKED WITH BULGUR

Using bulgur instead of rice makes the initial change of pace here. And then the apple juice–wine combo, poured over all, really turns the trick. If cilantro is not your thing, garnish with chopped scallions or parsley.

½ cup bulgur
2 teaspoons vegetable or olive oil
4 chicken thighs (about 1 pound total), skin and fat removed
Salt and freshly ground pepper to taste
¾ cup apple juice
¼ cup dry white wine
2 tablespoons chopped fresh cilantro

1. In a small bowl, combine bulgur with water to cover. Allow bulgur to soak for 20 minutes, then drain and set aside.
2. Preheat oven to 350° F.
3. Heat oil in an ovenproof casserole. Season chicken with salt and pepper to taste and add to casserole. Cook over medium-high heat, turning chicken, until golden on all sides, about 5 minutes.
4. Add drained bulgur to chicken in casserole. Pour apple juice and wine over chicken and bulgur, cover, and bake for 30 to 45 minutes or until chicken is tender and cooked through.
5. Garnish with cilantro and serve.

SERVES 4

Per serving: 190 calories; 16.0 grams protein; 19.5 grams carbohydrates; 5.3 grams fat; 57 milligrams cholesterol; 65 milligrams sodium (without salting).

CHICKEN BASQUAISE

Since thieves once roamed the Pyrénées Mountains that create the jagged fence between France and Spain, the story is that the original recipe for this chicken dish began: First, you steal a chicken . . . Untrue? Of course. But this highly seasoned, low fat meal-in-one is for real.

2 teaspoons olive oil
1 3-pound chicken, skin and fat removed, quartered
   Salt and freshly ground pepper to taste
1 cup rice
1½ cups Low Fat Chicken Stock (page 3) or canned low sodium broth
4 tomatoes, peeled and quartered
1 jalapeño or hot cherry pepper, cored, seeded, and diced (wear gloves)

1. Preheat oven to 350° F.
2. Heat oil in a large nonstick skillet. Add chicken and cook over medium-high heat for about 10 minutes or until chicken is browned on all sides. Do not cook through.
3. Transfer chicken to an ovenproof casserole with a cover and season to taste.
4. Add rice to skillet and cook over low heat, stirring, for 2 minutes. Spoon rice over and around chicken. Pour in stock and arrange tomato sections and hot pepper on rice.
5. Cover and bake for 30 to 45 minutes or until

chicken and rice are cooked through. If necessary add more liquid, one or two tablespoons at a time. Bring casserole to the table and serve hot.

SERVES 4

Per serving: 400 calories; 40.0 grams protein; 43.0 grams carbohydrates; 7.6 grams fat; 117 milligrams cholesterol; 220 milligrams sodium (without salting).

CHILI-SPICED PICNIC DRUMSTICKS

Because it is so easy to handle, this dish is just the ticket for a picnic meal—but don't disregard it as an offering in your own dining room.

Serve it with a colorful mélange of crudités that are quick to prepare and simple to transport.

  8 chicken drumsticks (about 1 pound total), skin and
      fat removed
¹/₄ cup fresh lime juice
  1 tablespoon chili powder, or to taste
      Salt to taste
      Vegetable oil cooking spray

1. Preheat oven to 375° F.

2. Moisten drumsticks with lime juice, season with chili powder, and sprinkle with salt if you wish.

3. Coat a shallow baking pan with cooking spray. Place drumsticks in pan and bake for 30 to 45 minutes, turning drumsticks every 15 minutes, until brown, tender, and cooked through. Remove from oven and let cool to room temperature before serving.

SERVES 4
Per serving: 90 calories; 13.0 grams protein; 2.5 grams carbohydrates; 3.2 grams fat; 48 milligrams cholesterol; 75 milligrams sodium (without salting).

ROSEMARY CHICKEN
BAKED ON A CELERY BED

Today's home cooks are really the new pioneers who search out ways of using natural seasonings to bring out the big flavors without the fat. By baking or roasting vegetables, such as the celery in my recipe below, the flavors become concentrated, making added fat unnecessary. The addition of herbs will add enormous dimension.

Serve with kasha, grits, polenta, or rice and a simple mixed greens salad.

2 bunches celery
1 teaspoon celery seeds
1 3-pound chicken, skin and fat removed, cut into 8 pieces
1 teaspoon fresh rosemary
  Salt and freshly ground pepper to taste
2 cups Low Fat Chicken Stock (page 3) or canned low sodium broth
¼ cup dry white vermouth
1 tablespoon chopped fresh parsley

1. Preheat oven to 350° F.

2. Discard celery leaves, wash celery and remove strings with a vegetable peeler. Chop celery into ½-inch slices. Toss with celery seeds and spoon mixture onto bottom of a roasting pan.

3. Season chicken with rosemary, salt and pepper and place on top of celery.

4. Heat stock and vermouth in a small saucepan to a simmer. Pour over chicken and bake for about 1½ hours or until chicken is tender, lightly browned, and cooked through. Baste every 15 minutes.

5. Remove chicken to a platter and keep warm. Using a slotted spoon, transfer celery to a serving platter. Place chicken pieces on top, moisten with pan juices, garnish with parsley, and serve.

SERVES 4

Per serving: 230 calories; 36.5 grams protein; 6.0 grams carbohydrates; 6.5 grams fat; 118 milligrams cholesterol; 250 milligrams sodium (without salting).

BAKED CHICKEN BASIL
WITH PARMESAN

The addition of low fat Parmesan cheese pushes up the flavors of this chicken, tomato, and basil combo, producing a dish that is bright and exciting without being heavy. Terrific with spaghetti squash.

1 pound skinless and boneless chicken breasts, fat removed
2 teaspoons olive oil
3 cloves garlic, minced
3/4 cup chopped fresh basil leaves
4 plum tomatoes, diced
1/4 cup dry white wine
1 teaspoon balsamic vinegar
Salt and freshly ground pepper to taste
1 1/2 tablespoons grated low fat Parmesan cheese

1. Preheat oven to 350° F. Place chicken breasts in a single layer in an ovenproof casserole or baking pan and set aside.

2. Heat oil in a small nonstick skillet. Add garlic and stir over high heat for 1 minute. Add all remaining ingredients, except cheese, to skillet and cook, stirring, for 10 minutes.

3. Spoon skillet ingredients over chicken and bake for 20 minutes. Sprinkle with grated cheese and bake an additional 10 minutes or until chicken is tender and cooked through.

Per serving: 185 calories; 29.0 grams protein; 7.0 grams carbohydrates; 4.5 grams fat; 66 milligrams cholesterol; 130 milligrams sodium (without salting).

BARBECUE-BAKED CHICKEN

Here, the chicken is baked in a barbecue sauce that can also be used to grill, broil, or barbecue the bird.

1 teaspoon vegetable or peanut oil
1 cup canned no-salt-added tomato sauce
1/2 cup cider vinegar
2 tablespoons fresh lemon juice
1 medium onion, finely minced
2 teaspoons chili powder
2 teaspoons dry mustard
2 teaspoons brown sugar
Salt and freshly ground pepper to taste
1 3-pound chicken, skin and fat removed, quartered

1. Combine all ingredients, except chicken, in a small saucepan. Bring to a boil, then reduce heat and simmer gently for 10 minutes. Remove from heat and let cool slightly.

2. Place chicken in a large bowl. Spoon sauce over chicken, covering all sides, cover bowl, and refrigerate for 45 minutes.

3. Preheat oven to 400° F.

4. Place chicken, meat side up, in a shallow baking pan in a single layer. Spoon half the sauce over chicken. Bake, basting with remaining sauce occasionally, for 45 minutes to 1 hour or until chicken is tender and cooked through.

5. Transfer chicken to a heated platter, spoon sauce from pan over chicken, and serve.

SERVES 4

Per serving: 255 calories; 36.5 grams protein; 11.5 grams carbohydrates; 6.8 grams fat; 115 milligrams cholesterol; 160 milligrams sodium (without salting).

BAKED CHICKEN THIGHS WITH ORANGE-MUSTARD-HONEY SAUCE

This is the kind of dish I keep hoping will have something left over because it tastes even better the next day. For that reason alone, I usually make more than is called for in the recipe. Nifty with a slaw made with thinly sliced cabbage, carrot, and red bell pepper.

2 teaspoons vegetable oil
4 chicken thighs (about 1 pound total), skin and fat
    removed
¾ cup orange juice
1 tablespoon Dijon mustard
2 teaspoons honey
    Salt and freshly ground pepper to taste
1 large seedless orange, peeled and cut into horizontal
    slices

1. Preheat oven to 350° F.

2. Heat oil in a medium nonstick skillet. Add chicken and brown over high heat, turning from side to side. Remove chicken thighs from skillet and place in a baking pan.

3. Combine orange juice, mustard, and honey in a small bowl and stir until well blended. Spoon mixture over chicken and bake for 45 minutes to 1 hour or until tender. Baste occasionally and turn chicken thighs after 30 minutes.

4. Transfer chicken to a heated serving platter, spoon on any sauce from baking pan, and serve garnished with orange slices.

SERVES 4

Per serving: 155 calories; 14.5 grams protein; 11.5 grams carbohydrates; 5.4 grams fat; 57 milligrams cholesterol; 175 milligrams sodium (without salting).

GRATIN OF CHICKEN AND BROCCOLI

I like to serve this one-dish meal right from the casserole in which it has been cooked. Accompany it with a salad of baby lettuces and other crisp greens such as watercress.

1 small bunch broccoli
1/2 cup Low Fat Chicken Stock (page 3) or canned low
    sodium broth
2 large shallots, finely minced
    Salt and freshly ground pepper to taste
1 skinless and boneless chicken breast (about 1 pound),
    fat removed and split
    Egg substitute equal to 2 eggs
3/4 cup low fat (1%) milk
1 tablespoon chopped fresh parsley
1/2 cup bread crumbs, made from 1 slice dry whole
    wheat or white bread
2 tablespoons grated low fat Parmesan or Romano
    cheese, optional
    Vegetable oil cooking spray

1. Break broccoli into florets. In a medium saucepan, cook florets in boiling water to cover for 2 minutes. Drain and set aside.

2. Combine stock, shallots, and salt and pepper in a large skillet and bring to a simmer. Add chicken, reduce heat to low, cover, and simmer for 15 to 20 minutes or until chicken is just cooked through. Remove

chicken from skillet and set aside to cool. Reserve pan juices.

3. Preheat oven to 350° F.

4. Coarsely chop broccoli and transfer to a large bowl. Coarsely chop chicken and add to broccoli. Stir in pan juices.

5. Whisk together egg substitute and milk and pour over chicken-broccoli combination. Add parsley, bread crumbs, and cheese if desired, and mix until all ingredients are combined. Taste and adjust seasonings if needed.

6. Spoon chicken-broccoli mixture into a shallow, ovenproof casserole lightly coated with cooking spray. Bake for about 30 minutes or until top is brown and all ingredients are simmering. Remove from oven and let stand 1 minute before serving.

SERVES 4

Per serving: 220 calories; 35.0 grams protein; 11.0 grams carbohydrates; 3.9 grams fat; 69 milligrams cholesterol; 250 milligrams sodium (without salting).

STUFFED AND ROASTED SQUAB

A squab is a small chicken, about one pound in weight. In France this small bird is called *poussin*, and some butchers in America also prefer to call these delicate birds by their French name.

The trick in preparing squab is to place the stuffing under the bird's skin rather than in the cavity. Not only does the stuffing flavor the bird and keep the breast moist, it also causes the bird to plump as it roasts, and the result is an appealing and delicious dish.

2 squab (about 1 pound each), split
4 thin slices white bread, crusts removed
2 shallots, quartered
1 clove garlic, quartered
  Egg substitute equal to 1 egg
1/4 cup fresh parsley sprigs
  Salt and freshly ground pepper to taste
1 1/2 cups Low Fat Chicken Stock (page 3) or canned low
       sodium broth
  Paprika to taste

1. Preheat oven to 375° F.
2. Very carefully loosen the skin over the breasts of the birds and set aside.
3. Combine bread, shallots, garlic, egg substitute, parsley, and salt and pepper in a food processor and process briefly, until coarsely ground.
4. Using a small spoon, insert stuffing between skin

and breast meat of the birds. Place birds, skin side up, in a large roasting pan or ovenproof casserole that has a cover.

5. Heat stock in a small saucepan to a simmer and pour over birds. Sprinkle with paprika.

6. Cover and roast for 30 minutes, basting after 15 minutes. Remove cover, baste again, and roast uncovered, basting after 15 minutes, for 30 to 45 minutes, or until birds are tender and well browned.

SERVES 4

Per serving: 240 calories; 23.5 grams protein; 11.0 grams carbohydrates; 11.0 grams fat; 68 milligrams cholesterol; 190 milligrams sodium (without salting).

ROASTED BREAST OF TURKEY AND VEGETABLES

Boneless breast of turkey is easy to prepare and a delight to serve. After it's cooked it can be thinly sliced and served either hot or cold.

This is perfect party food, and if there are leftovers the meat is a delicious addition to sandwiches or salads.

1 large red bell pepper, seeded, cut into 6 slices
1 large green bell pepper, seeded, cut into 6 slices
3 small red jacket potatoes, halved
1 large onion, cut into 6 wedges
2 teaspoons olive oil
1 teaspoon dried rosemary
Salt and freshly ground pepper to taste
1½ pound skinless and boneless turkey breast, in one piece
1½ cups Low Fat Turkey-Herb Stock (page 5), Low Fat Chicken Stock (page 3), or canned low sodium chicken broth
12 small cherry tomatoes
4 sprigs fresh parsley

1. Preheat oven to 350° F.

2. In a medium mixing bowl, combine bell peppers, potatoes, onion, 1 teaspoon oil, rosemary, salt and pepper, and toss lightly.

3. Place turkey in center of a medium roasting pan, season with salt and pepper if desired, and spread re-

maining oil over turkey. Strew vegetables around turkey, and pour stock over vegetables.

4. Roast for about 45 minutes to 1 hour or until turkey and vegetables are tender and cooked through.

5. Transfer turkey to a cutting board and let stand for about 2 minutes, then cut into thin slices. Arrange slices on a heated platter, surround turkey with vegetables, spoon pan juices over all, and serve garnished with cherry tomatoes and parsley sprigs.

SERVES 6
Per serving: 205 calories; 30.0 grams protein; 14.0 grams carbohydrates; 3.2 grams fat; 72 milligrams cholesterol; 90 milligrams sodium (without salting).

THE MAIN DISH:
BRAISED AND LIGHTLY SAUTÉED

CHICKEN SAUTÉ
WITH BALSAMIC VINEGAR

In this simple recipe, a marvelously complex flavor develops by combining homemade chicken stock with balsamic vinegar. Garlic and plum tomatoes are added to produce a truly memorable entrée of chicken with little fuss . . . and a lot of taste!

I like to eat this with polenta or sweet potatoes and a quick-steamed vegetable, such as green beans, spinach, or cauliflower.

> 1 teaspoon olive oil
> 1 3-pound chicken, skin and fat removed, cut into 8 pieces
> Salt and freshly ground pepper to taste
> 2 cloves garlic, minced
> 4 plum tomatoes, chopped
> 2 tablespoons balsamic vinegar or to taste
> 1/2 cup Low Fat Chicken Stock (page 3) or canned low sodium broth

1. Heat oil in a large nonstick skillet or Dutch oven. Add chicken, season to taste with salt and pepper, and sauté until just golden, about 5 minutes on each side.

2. Add garlic and tomatoes to chicken in skillet and continue sautéing for 2 minutes.

3. Add vinegar and stock and bring to a simmer. Cover and cook over low heat for about 45 minutes or until chicken is tender and cooked through. Transfer to a heated platter and serve.

SERVES 4

Per serving: 235 calories; 36.5 grams protein; 6.5 grams carbohydrates; 6.7 grams fat; 116 milligrams cholesterol; 150 milligrams sodium (without salting).

CHICKEN BREAST BRAISED WITH ORANGE AND CARDAMOM

A member of the ginger family, cardamom has a pungent aroma and a warm, spicy-sweet flavor. Here, I've combined it with a jolt of hot sauce, stock, and orange juice for a spunky, not-your-ordinary breast of chicken entrée.

I serve this dish with fragrant brown basmati rice and cucumber raita (cucumber in a light yogurt-based sauce).

1 pound skinless and boneless chicken breasts, fat
    removed, cut into 4 pieces
  Salt and freshly ground pepper to taste
2 cups Low Fat Chicken Stock (page 3) or canned low
    sodium broth
1 teaspoon hot pepper sauce
1/2 teaspoon ground cardamom or to taste
2 teaspoons cornstarch
1/2 cup orange juice
1 medium seedless orange, peeled and cut into 4
    horizontal slices

1. Season chicken and place in a skillet in one layer.
2. Combine stock, hot pepper sauce, and cardamom in a small saucepan. Bring to a simmer and pour over chicken in a large skillet. Cover and simmer over low heat for about 25 minutes or until chicken is cooked through.
3. Combine cornstarch and orange juice in a small

bowl. Mix thoroughly and pour over chicken in skillet. Add orange slices and cook, stirring, until sauce thickens slightly.

4. Transfer chicken, sauce, and orange slices to a heated platter and serve.

SERVES 4

Per serving: 165 calories; 27.0 grams protein; 9.5 grams carbohydrates; 2.2 grams fat; 67 milligrams cholesterol; 125 milligrams sodium (without salting).

BRAISED CHICKEN BREAST WITH GRAPES AND OLIVES OVER RICE

Cardamom is an unusual spice in that it goes equally well with meats and fruits. This may account for the fact that it's used extensively in the seemingly opposite cuisines of Scandinavians and East Indians.

In the recipe that follows, I use the warm, spicy-sweet flavor of the cardamom as a conduit between grapes and olives to make this unusual but satisfying entrée.

1½ cups Low Fat Chicken Stock (page 3) or canned low sodium broth
1 pound skinless and boneless chicken breasts, fat removed
¼ cup chopped fresh parsley
Salt and freshly ground pepper to taste
¼ cup dry vermouth
½ teaspoon ground cardamom
1 cup red seedless grapes, halved
6 black pitted olives, sliced
2 cups cooked hot rice

1. Heat stock to a simmer in a large skillet. Add chicken, parsley, and salt and pepper to taste. Cover and cook over low heat until chicken is tender and cooked through, about 15 minutes. Remove chicken from skillet and set aside.

2. Add vermouth and cardamom to skillet and bring to a simmer. Cover and cook for 5 minutes.

3. Cut chicken into thin slices and return to skillet. Add grapes and olives and cook about 2 minutes or until all ingredients are thoroughly heated.

4. Place rice on a heated platter and spoon chicken with grapes and sauce over rice. Serve hot.

SERVES 4

Per serving: 290 calories; 29.5 grams protein; 35.5 grams carbohydrates; 3.2 grams fat; 67 milligrams cholesterol; 165 milligrams sodium (without salting).

INDONESIAN-STYLE CHICKEN WITH BOK CHOY

Bok choy (also called Chinese mustard cabbage) resembles a cross between celery and green Swiss chard. In its raw state, the leaves have a slightly sharp tang while the stalks are not as bitter; cooking, however, turns the leaves milder and the stalks sweeter. Bok choy is great for slaws, soups, and dishes like this highly seasoned Indonesian-inspired chicken.

If bok choy is unavailable, Napa cabbage, which is less assertive, may be substituted.

1 teaspoon vegetable oil
1 pound skinless and boneless chicken breasts, fat removed, cubed
3 cloves garlic, pressed
1 tablespoon minced fresh ginger
1 small onion, diced
1 small head bok choy (about 1 pound), trimmed, cut into thin 1-inch pieces
Juice of 1 lemon
2 teaspoons low sodium soy sauce
1 cup Low Fat Chicken Stock (page 3) or canned low sodium broth
1/2 teaspoon hot pepper sauce or to taste
1 teaspoon brown sugar
1/2 teaspoon ground turmeric

1. Heat oil in a large nonstick skillet. Add chicken and cook over medium heat, stirring, for about 5

minutes or until lightly browned and cooked through. Remove chicken from skillet and set aside.

2. Add garlic, ginger, onion, and bok choy to skillet and cook, stirring, for 2 minutes. Add all remaining ingredients to skillet and reduce heat. Cover and cook over low heat for about 5 minutes or until bok choy is crisp-tender.

3. Return chicken to skillet. Mix to combine ingredients and heat through. Transfer to a heated platter and serve.

SERVES 4
Per serving: 170 calories; 28.0 grams protein; 7.5 grams carbohydrates; 3.3 grams fat; 66 milligrams cholesterol; 265 milligrams sodium (without salting).

CHICKEN WITH PLUMS AND TANGERINES OVER FETTUCCINE

A sweet and colorful dish that's always festive and always a hit. Almost any pasta—linguine, spaghetti, small shells, egg noodles—will work well here.

1 pound skinless and boneless chicken breasts, fat
    removed
1 cup low sodium tomato juice
    Salt and freshly ground pepper to taste
1 cup orange juice, preferably fresh-squeezed
1 tablespoon fresh lemon juice
1 tablespoon honey or to taste
2 teaspoons peanut or vegetable oil
1/4 teaspoon ground nutmeg
1/4 teaspoon ground cinnamon
1/2 pound fettuccine
2 fresh plums, pitted and sliced
1 tangerine, peeled, pitted, and sectioned
1 tablespoon cornstarch
2 tablespoons cold water
    Parsley for garnish

1. Combine chicken, tomato juice, and salt and pepper to taste in a large skillet. Cover and bring to a boil, then reduce heat to low and simmer gently, turning chicken once, for 15 to 20 minutes or until chicken is cooked through. Transfer chicken to a cutting board; cut into 1-inch cubes and set aside.

2. Combine orange and lemon juices, honey, and oil

in a large saucepan and stir over medium heat until thoroughly blended. Cover and reduce heat and simmer for 5 minutes.

3. While sauce simmers, cook fettuccine in a large pot of boiling water until al dente.

4. Add plums and oranges to orange-honey mixture in saucepan. Stir over medium high heat for 5 minutes. In a small bowl, dissolve cornstarch in water and add to sauce and fruits. Stir until simmering and thickened. Add chicken and simmer for 1 minute or until chicken is heated through.

5. Drain fettuccine and transfer to a heated serving bowl or platter. Spoon chicken, fruit, and sauce over pasta, garnish with parsley, and serve immediately.

SERVES 4

Per serving: 430 calories; 34.5 grams protein; 60.5 grams carbohydrates; 5.2 grams fat; 65 milligrams cholesterol; 85 milligrams sodium (without salting).

CITRUS CHICKEN

I adore the sparkling taste the chicken gets from the thickened orange and lime sauce. Serve with a salad of grated carrots and bean sprouts for added color and textural interest.

    2 teaspoons olive oil
    1 3-pound chicken, skin and fat removed, cut into 8
        pieces
    Salt and freshly ground pepper to taste
1 1/2 cups orange juice
    1 seedless orange, peeled and coarsely chopped
    2 teaspoons minced orange peel
    1 lime, peeled and coarsely chopped
    2 teaspoons minced lime peel
1 1/2 tablespoons sugar or to taste
    2 teaspoons cornstarch
    1/4 cup water

1. Heat oil in a large nonstick skillet. Add chicken in one layer. Season to taste and sauté over medium heat, turning chicken to brown on all sides, for 30 to 45 minutes or until cooked through.

2. While chicken cooks, combine 1 cup orange juice, orange and orange peel, lime and lime peel, and sugar in a small saucepan and simmer, covered, over low heat for 15 minutes.

3. When chicken is cooked, remove from skillet and keep warm. Pour remaining orange juice into skillet and stir over high heat for 2 minutes. Add contents of

saucepan to skillet and cook, stirring, for an additional minute.

4. Combine cornstarch and water in a small bowl. Mix well and add to fruit sauce in skillet. Cook, stirring over low heat, until sauce thickens slightly.

5. Transfer chicken to a heated platter and pour sauce over chicken before serving.

SERVES 4

Per serving: 285 calories; 36.5 grams protein; 17.5 grams carbohydrates; 7.8 grams fat; 115 milligrams cholesterol; 130 milligrams sodium (without salting).

CHICKEN WITH MUSHROOMS AND ZUCCHINI

Easy to put together, and easy on the fat and calories—all that's needed is some polenta or rice to round out dinner.

2 teaspoons olive oil
¼ pound mushrooms, wiped clean and thinly sliced
2 small zucchini, thinly sliced
1 pound skinless and boneless chicken breasts, fat removed
  Juice of 1 large lemon
  Salt and freshly ground pepper to taste
1 tablespoon finely chopped fresh coriander leaves (cilantro) or Italian parsley

1. Heat oil in a large nonstick skillet. Add mushrooms and zucchini and cook over medium-high heat, stirring occasionally, for about 2 minutes. Using a slotted spoon, remove vegetables from skillet and set aside.

2. Place chicken in skillet in one layer and sauté over medium-high heat, turning to brown lightly on both sides, for 5 to 10 minutes or until cooked through. Remove chicken with a slotted spatula and keep warm on a heated serving platter.

3. Add lemon juice, salt, and pepper to skillet and stir over high heat for 30 seconds. Pour contents of skillet over chicken. Top with reserved vegetables,

garnish with cilantro or parsley, and serve immediately.

SERVES 4

Per serving: 155 calories; 27.5 grams protein; 3.0 grams carbohydrates; 3.8 grams fat; 65 milligrams cholesterol; 75 milligrams sodium (without salting).

NEAPOLITAN COUNTRY-STYLE CHICKEN

This is a greatly fat-reduced version of a southern Italian dish, alternately known as "Farmer's Chicken," "Peasant's Chicken," or "Chicken Contadina," which usually contains a great deal of olive oil.

Complete this one-dish meal with a salad of crisp seasonal greens tossed with fresh lemon juice and a bottle of Chianti.

2 teaspoons olive oil
2 medium baking potatoes, peeled and cubed
1 large onion, sliced
1 large green bell pepper, cut into strips
1 large stalk celery, diced
1 clove garlic, minced
1 pound skinless and boneless chicken breasts, fat removed, thinly sliced
1 cup Low Fat Chicken Stock (page 3) or canned low sodium broth
2 medium tomatoes, chopped
$1/4$ teaspoon hot pepper flakes, optional
Salt and freshly ground pepper to taste

1. Heat oil in a large nonstick skillet. Add potatoes to skillet, and cook over medium-high heat for 10 minutes, turning potatoes to brown as they cook.

2. Add onion, bell pepper, and celery to skillet. Lower heat slightly and cook for an additional 5 min-

utes. Add garlic and chicken. Stir gently to combine and cook for an additional 3 minutes.

3. Add remaining ingredients. Cover and cook over low heat, stirring occasionally, for 15 minutes or until potatoes and chicken are tender and cooked through. Transfer all ingredients from skillet to a platter and serve immediately.

SERVES 4

Per serving: 235 calories; 29.0 grams protein; 20.5 grams carbohydrates; 4.5 grams fat; 65 milligrams cholesterol; 110 milligrams sodium (without salting).

CHICKEN LAYERED WITH SPINACH AND PINE NUTS

Pine nuts, or "pignoli," have long been a staple in the Italian and Native American kitchens, and I've used them here for both their taste and texture.

1 pound spinach
2 teaspoons olive oil
1 tablespoon pine nuts
   Salt and freshly ground pepper to taste
8 pieces chicken cutlets (about 1 pound total), pounded
   thin
1 red bell pepper, diced

1. Wash spinach thoroughly and break off and discard tough stems. Drain and spin dry. Chop coarsely.

2. Heat 1 teaspoon oil in a large nonstick skillet. Add spinach and cover. Cook for about 3 minutes or until spinach has wilted. Add pine nuts and salt and pepper to spinach, and continue cooking for another 3 or 4 minutes or until liquid has evaporated. Transfer to a heated covered dish and keep warm.

3. Heat remaining teaspoon oil in skillet. Season chicken and add to skillet in one layer. Sauté over medium-high heat, turning to brown lightly, for about 5 minutes or until chicken is cooked.

4. Place half the chicken on a heated serving platter, top with spinach, and cover with remaining pieces of chicken. Garnish with diced red pepper and serve.

SERVES 4

Per serving: 180 calories; 29.0 grams protein; 4.5 grams carbohydrates; 5.3 grams fat; 65 milligrams cholesterol; 150 milligrams sodium (without salting).

CHICKEN SCALLOPINE WITH BUTTON MUSHROOMS AND SHERRY

This is a dish that is traditionally prepared with veal. But I have found that it is just as tasty with chicken cutlets pounded into scallopine, and far lower in fat and cholesterol.

½ pound button mushrooms, wiped clean
½ cup Low Fat Chicken Stock (page 3) or canned low sodium broth
¼ teaspoon freshly ground pepper
Paprika to taste
2 tablespoons dry sherry
1 pound chicken cutlets, pounded thin
Salt and freshly ground pepper to taste
1 tablespoon all-purpose flour
1 teaspoon olive oil
¼ cup watercress sprigs

1. Combine mushrooms, stock, pepper, and paprika in a small saucepan. Cover and bring to a simmer. Cook for 3 minutes. Add sherry and continue cooking until mushrooms are just tender. Remove from heat and set aside.

2. Season chicken with salt and pepper. Place in a paper bag with flour and shake until chicken is lightly coated with flour. Remove from bag and shake off any excess flour.

3. Heat oil in a large nonstick skillet. Add chicken in

one layer and sauté over medium-high heat for 4 or 5 minutes or until chicken is done and lightly browned on both sides. Transfer chicken to a platter and keep warm.

4. Heat mushrooms and sauce until just simmering. Spoon sauce over chicken, garnish with watercress, and serve.

SERVES 4

Per serving: 160 calories; 27.5 grams protein; 5.0 grams carbohydrates; 3.0 grams fat; 65 milligrams cholesterol; 85 milligrams sodium (without salting).

CHICKEN AND SWEET PEPPER STRIPS WITH GINGER AND ARUGULA

Whether it's called "rocket," "rugula," "rucola," or "arugula," I love it! For me, nothing can beat this bitterish, aromatic salad green with its unique peppery-mustard flavor. When cooked briefly, it's a happy surprise. Sometimes I use it with pasta instead of basil. And I add it to dishes, such as the one described below, for its distinctive taste and rich color. Arugula is also loaded with beta-carotene, vitamin C, and calcium.

1 tablespoon olive oil

1 medium red onion, cut in half and thinly sliced

1 clove garlic, minced

2 tablespoons minced fresh ginger

1 small red bell pepper, trimmed and cut into 1/2-inch strips

1 small green bell pepper, trimmed and cut into 1/2-inch strips

Salt and freshly ground pepper to taste

3/4 pound skinless and boneless chicken breasts, fat removed, cut into 1/2-inch strips

2 teaspoons low sodium soy sauce

1 cup arugula leaves

1 tablespoon fine flour

1/4 cup Low Fat Chicken Stock (page 3) or canned low sodium chicken broth

1. Heat oil in a large nonstick skillet. Add onion and cook over medium heat, stirring frequently, for 3 minutes.

2. Add garlic, ginger, and bell peppers to skillet and cook, stirring, for 3 minutes. Season to taste with salt and pepper and add chicken strips and soy sauce. Reduce heat to low and cook, stirring frequently, for 5 minutes.

3. Add arugula to skillet, raise heat to medium-high and cook, stirring, for 2 minutes.

4. Dissolve flour in stock and add to skillet. Cook for about 1 minute or until chicken is tender and ingredients are heated throughout. Taste and adjust seasonings, if necessary, and serve.

SERVES 4

Per serving: 160 calories; 21.0 grams protein; 8.5 grams carbohydrates; 4.8 grams fat; 49 milligrams cholesterol; 165 milligrams sodium (without salting).

SKILLET CHICKEN WITH SWEET-AND-SOUR CABBAGE

This is a kind of *un*stuffed cabbage with chicken—and a kick of cayenne. The chicken is cooked on top of the sweetened-and-soured cabbage, imparting that particular flavor throughout. Then, tart Granny Smith apple sections are served with it to further extend the concept. Delicious, absolutely delicious!

    2 teaspoons vegetable oil
    1 3-pound chicken, skin and fat removed, cut into 8
        pieces
    3/4 cup apple juice
    1 small head cabbage (about 1 pound), coarsely
        chopped
    1 tablespoon brown sugar
    1 tablespoon cider vinegar
    1/8 teaspoon cayenne pepper or to taste
        Salt to taste
    1 Granny Smith apple

1. Heat oil in a large nonstick skillet. Add chicken and sauté over high heat for about 5 minutes on all sides or until lightly browned.

2. Add apple juice to skillet, reduce heat to medium and simmer for 5 minutes. Using a slotted spoon, remove chicken from skillet and set aside.

3. Add cabbage, sugar, vinegar, cayenne pepper, and salt to skillet. Cook, stirring, for about 2 minutes.

4. Place chicken pieces on top of cabbage in skillet.

Cover, reduce heat to very low, and cook for 30 to 45 minutes or until chicken is tender.

5. Remove chicken from skillet. Spoon a bed of cabbage on a heated serving platter, arrange chicken over cabbage and spoon any pan juices over all. Core apple and cut into 8 wedges; garnish with apple sections and serve.

SERVES 4

Per serving: 290 calories; 36.5 grams protein; 19.0 grams carbohydrates; 7.7 grams fat; 115 milligrams cholesterol; 145 milligrams sodium (without salting).

TURKEY, LEEKS, AND ARTICHOKES BRAISED IN GARLICKY TOMATO SAUCE

Commercially packaged artichoke hearts come from tiny whole artichokes that have almost no fuzzy "choke." Not only is the artichoke delectable, it is also a source of vitamin C and dietary fiber, and I always keep some around for a quick, tempting meal or snack. Try this artichoke, turkey, and leek dish over pasta of any kind, or over couscous, rice, or any other grain.

   4 cloves garlic
   2 teaspoons olive oil
   4 turkey cutlets (about 3/4 pound total)
   2 leeks, white and tender greens, well-rinsed and cut
      crosswise into 1/2-inch slices
   2 large cloves garlic, thinly sliced
   1 14-ounce can artichoke hearts, drained, rinsed, and
      cut in half
   1 cup canned low sodium tomato sauce
   1 tablespoon red wine vinegar
   1 tablespoon chopped fresh Italian parsley
   1 teaspoon dried oregano
      Salt and freshly ground pepper to taste

1. Cut 2 garlic cloves into very thin slices and set aside. Press remaining 2 cloves garlic and set aside.

2. Heat 1 teaspoon oil in a large nonstick skillet. Add turkey and cook over high heat for 1 or 2 min-

---

utes on each side or until golden. Reduce heat to medium. Remove turkey from skillet and set aside.

3. Heat remaining teaspoon oil in skillet and add sliced garlic and leeks. Cook, stirring, for 2 minutes.

4. Return turkey to skillet, add pressed garlic and add all remaining ingredients and bring to a simmer. Reduce heat to very low and simmer gently, uncovered, spooning sauce over turkey and artichokes occasionally, for 15 minutes or until turkey is cooked through (if too much liquid evaporates, add a little water).

5. Arrange turkey and artichokes on a heated serving platter, spoon sauce over all, and serve.

SERVES 4

Per serving: 180 calories; 24.0 grams protein; 14.0 grams carbohydrates; 3.3 grams fat; 54 milligrams cholesterol; 240 milligrams sodium (without salting).

TURKEY IN CURRY-GINGER SAUCE WITH MANGO AND KIWI

The sweetness of the mango contrasted with the semi-tart kiwi acts as a chutney for this curry-flavored dish. If mango and kiwi don't suit you, try whatever fruits you prefer.

1 teaspoon olive oil
1 pound turkey breast cutlets
Salt and freshly ground pepper to taste
1 cup Low Fat Chicken Stock (page 3) or canned low
    sodium broth
1 teaspoon curry powder
1 teaspoon ground ginger
1 ripe mango, peeled and cut into chunks
2 kiwi fruit, peeled and sliced horizontally

1. Heat oil in a large nonstick skillet. Season turkey and add to skillet in one layer. Sauté over medium-high heat, turning once, for about 10 minutes or until lightly browned and tender. Transfer turkey to a platter.

2. Add stock, curry powder, and ginger to skillet. Cook over medium-high heat until reduced by half. Return turkey to skillet and heat through.

3. Arrange mango and kiwi on the perimeter of a platter. Place turkey cutlets in center and spoon sauce over turkey before serving.

Per serving: 200 calories; 29.0 grams protein; 15.5 grams carbohydrates; 2.6 grams fat; 72 milligrams cholesterol; 75 milligrams sodium (without salting).

TURKEY CUTLETS
IN TARRAGON WINE SAUCE

Fabled in Spanish, Italian, and most notably French cookery, tarragon sauce is classically made with butter and heavy cream. In this recipe, by eliminating all but a smidgeon of fat, and instead using fresh lemon juice and wine to deglaze the pan in which the turkey has been cooked, you'll produce a superb and guilt-free dish.

    4 turkey breast cutlets (about 1 pound)
    3 tablespoons all-purpose flour
      Salt and freshly ground pepper to taste
    2 teaspoons olive oil
    ³/₄ cup dry white wine
    1 tablespoon fresh lemon juice
    1 teaspoon dried tarragon
    1 lemon, thinly sliced

1. Pound turkey breasts between wax paper or plastic wrap to a thickness of about ¹/₄ inch.

2. On a plate combine flour with salt and pepper. Dredge cutlets in seasoned flour and shake off any excess.

3. Heat oil in a nonstick skillet large enough to hold cutlets in one layer (or cook in 2 batches). Add cutlets and cook over medium heat for 2 to 3 minutes on each side or until lightly browned and almost cooked through. Transfer cutlets to a platter.

4. Add wine, lemon juice, and tarragon to skillet

and bring to a boil. Reduce heat to medium-high and stir for 1 minute or until liquid is slightly reduced.

5. Return cutlets to skillets and cook 1 minute on each side or until cooked through.

6. Transfer cutlets to a heated serving platter. Spoon sauce from skillet over cutlets, and serve garnished with lemon slices.

SERVES 4
Per serving: 170 calories; 28.5 grams protein; 6.5 grams carbohydrates; 3.4 grams fat; 71 milligrams cholesterol; 60 milligrams sodium (without salting).

STIR-FRIED TURKEY
CALIFORNIA STYLE

No place beats California for setting trends in new food combinations, and I've adapted some Left Coast and Far East ideas that fit right into our reduced-fat scheme of things.

It is imperative to have all raw foods and seasonings close at hand and ready for the quick cooking that stir-frying requires. Serve over or with brown rice or cellophane noodles with thinly sliced scallions.

> 2 teaspoons olive oil
> 1 pound skinless and boneless turkey breast, cubed
> 2 celery stalks, thinly sliced
> 2 cups shredded Napa cabbage
> 8 small red radishes, thinly sliced
> 2 teaspoons low sodium soy sauce
> 1 teaspoon sesame oil
> 1/4 teaspoon Szechuan pepper or hot red pepper flakes, or to taste
> 1/4 cup Low Fat Chicken Stock (page 3) or canned low sodium broth
> 1 tablespoon cornstarch
> 1/4 cup water
>   Salt and freshly ground pepper to taste

1. Heat oil in a large nonstick skillet. Add turkey, and cook, stirring, for 5 minutes.

2. Add celery, cabbage, radish, soy sauce, and ses-

ame oil to skillet. Cook, stirring, over medium-high heat for 4 to 5 minutes or until cabbage is wilted.

3. Add pepper and stock to skillet and continue cooking for 3 minutes.

4. Combine cornstarch and stock in a small bowl. Mix well and add to skillet. Cook, stirring, until sauce has thickened slightly. Season to taste and serve.

SERVES 4

Per serving: 180 calories; 28.5 grams protein; 5.5 grams carbohydrates; 4.7 grams fat; 72 milligrams cholesterol; 145 milligrams sodium (without salting).

THE MAIN DISH:
BROILED AND GRILLED

CHICKEN GRILLED WITH LEMON AND GREEN PEPPERCORNS

This is a dream come true: a streamlined version of my all-time bistro favorite steak *au poivre,* using chicken in place of beef. Serve with disks of roasted sweet potato and a salad of arugula and endive.

    1 3-pound chicken, skin and fat removed, quartered
    ½ cup fresh lemon juice
    2 tablespoons crushed green peppercorns
    2 teaspoons olive oil
    Salt
    Vegetable oil cooking spray

1. Place chicken in a shallow pan. Spoon on lemon juice and spread peppercorns over chicken, pressing in with fingers, then dribble oil over chicken and add salt. Cover and refrigerate for 3 to 4 hours, turning chicken pieces in marinade every 30 minutes.

2. Prepare grill or preheat broiler.

3. Coat grill or broiler pan with cooking spray. Arrange chicken pieces on grill or pan and cook 5 to 6 inches from heat, turning pieces and brushing occasionally with marinade, for about 45 minutes or until chicken is browned, tender, and cooked through.

SERVES 4

Per serving: 225 calories; 35.5 grams protein; 2.5 grams carbohydrates; 8.1 grams fat; 115 milligrams cholesterol; 130 milligrams sodium (without salting).

TANDOORI CHICKEN
WITH YOGURT-MINT SAUCE

This is the kind of Delhi that makes good heart-healthy sense. By marinating chicken in a tempting blend of seasoned yogurt, the chicken becomes more succulent as the flavor of the spices develop and penetrate the flesh. Accompany with broad noodles or basmati or texmati rice.

   1 cup nonfat plain yogurt
     Juice of 1 lime
   1 clove garlic, pressed
   1 teaspoon each: ground cumin and dried coriander
   1/2 teaspoon each: powdered ginger, turmeric, cardamom
   1/4 teaspoon cayenne or hot paprika, or to taste
     Salt to taste
   1 3-pound chicken, skin and fat removed, quartered

YOGURT-MINT SAUCE
   1 cup nonfat yogurt
   1/4 cup packed fresh mint leaves or 2 tablespoon dried
     crushed mint
     Juice of 1 lime
     Salt and freshly ground pepper to taste

1. Combine yogurt, lime juice, garlic, spices, and salt in a small bowl. Stir until ingredients are thoroughly blended.

2. Coat chicken with yogurt mixture, rubbing in

spices on all sides of chicken. Place chicken in large bowl, cover, and refrigerate for 8 hours or overnight.

3. Preheat broiler.

4. Remove chicken from marinade and place in a shallow baking pan. Broil 5 to 6 inches from heat, turning occasionally and brushing with any leftover marinade, for about 45 minutes or until chicken is cooked through.

5. While chicken broils, combine all sauce ingredients in a food processor and process until smoothly blended. Transfer to a serving bowl and refrigerate until chicken is cooked.

6. Serve hot chicken with sauce on the side.

SERVES 4

Per serving: 260 calories; 41.5 grams protein; 10.0 grams carbohydrates; 5.2 grams fat; 118 milligrams cholesterol; 215 milligrams sodium (without salting).

CHICKEN WITH SPINACH AND LEEKS

My light adaptation of Chicken Florentine combines leeks with wine- and lemon-scented spinach.

2 teaspoons vegetable or olive oil
4 chicken cutlets (about ³/₄ pound total), pounded thin
3 leeks, white and tender greens, rinsed and chopped
1 clove garlic, minced
¹/₂ cup Low Fat Chicken Stock (page 3) or canned low sodium broth
2 tablespoons white wine
2 teaspoons fresh lemon juice
1 pound spinach, rinsed, tough stems removed, chopped
    Salt and freshly ground pepper to taste
    Vegetable or olive oil cooking spray
4 thin slices low fat Swiss cheese (about 1 ounce)

1. Heat oil in a large nonstick skillet. Add chicken cutlets to skillet and cook over medium-high heat for about 2 minutes on each side or until lightly browned. Remove from skillet and set aside. Do not wipe skillet.

2. Preheat broiler.

3. Add leeks and garlic to skillet and cook over medium heat for 5 minutes, stirring frequently. Raise heat to high. Add stock, wine, and lemon juice and bring to a boil. Add spinach and salt and pepper to taste. Cook, stirring frequently, for about 10 minutes or until liquid is reduced by about half.

4. Using a slotted spoon, transfer spinach-leek mixture to individual shallow ovenproof dishes (or arrange mixture into four equal mounds in a large casserole) lightly coated with cooking spray. Top spinach-leek mixture with a chicken cutlet. Spoon sauce from skillet over chicken and top with a strip of cheese. Broil 4 to 5 inches from heat for about 5 minutes or until chicken is cooked through and cheese is melted. Serve immediately.

SERVES 4

Per serving: 190 calories; 24.5 grams protein; 10.0 grams carbohydrates; 6.2 grams fat; 54 milligrams cholesterol; 145 milligrams sodium (without salting).

GRILLED DRUMSTICKS AND SWEET POTATOES OVER RICE

I, for one, can live on sweet potatoes. Absolutely delicious in nearly every state but raw, these sweeties are loaded with vitamins C and A, and contain some potassium, fiber, iron, and calcium. Here they are grilled with drumsticks and served along with a hot marinade/sauce over nutritious brown rice for a memorable dinner.

>   1 cup canned no-salt-added tomato sauce
>   2 tablespoons red wine vinegar
>   2 teaspoons hot pepper sauce
>   2 teaspoons brown sugar
>   2 cloves garlic, pressed
>   Salt to taste
>   8 chicken drumsticks (about 1 pound total), skin and
>   fat removed
>   Vegetable oil cooking spray
>   4 long sweet potatoes, scrubbed and cut lengthwise in
>   half
>   2 cups cooked brown rice

1. Prepare grill or preheat broiler.

2. Combine tomato sauce, vinegar, hot sauce, sugar, garlic, and salt in a saucepan. Bring to a simmer and stir for 2 minutes. Set half the sauce aside and cover to keep warm.

3. Place drumsticks in a large bowl and spoon on

remaining tomato sauce mixture, turning drumsticks to coat all sides.

4. Coat grill or broiler rack with cooking spray. Remove chicken from marinade and place on grill about 6 inches from heat. Grill for 10 minutes.

5. Add potatoes and grill for an additional 20 to 30 minutes or until chicken and potatoes are tender and cooked through, turning chicken and potatoes to brown on all sides, and brushing with marinade.

6. Spoon rice on a heated serving platter, arrange drumsticks and sweet potatoes over rice, spoon reserved warm sauce over all, and serve.

SERVES 4

Per serving: 355 calories; 18.5 grams protein; 61.0 grams carbohydrates; 4.3 grams fat; 48 milligrams cholesterol; 130 milligrams sodium (without salting).

CHICKEN BROILED WITH LIME-CUMIN MARINADE

Cumin, with its aromatic, nutty-peppery flavor is complex and marries well with many foods. Here I've united it with other seasonings in an uncommonly tasty marinade for chicken. Team with couscous or barley and fava beans for a totally "today" kind of menu.

   3/4 cup fresh lime juice
    2 teaspoons vegetable oil
    2 cloves garlic, pressed
1 1/2 teaspoons ground cumin
   1/2 teaspoon dried oregano
      Salt to taste
    1 3-pound chicken, skin and fat removed, quartered
      Vegetable oil cooking spray
    1 tablespoon finely chopped fresh cilantro

1. Combine lime juice, oil, garlic, cumin, oregano, and salt in a small bowl and mix thoroughly. Spoon marinade over chicken, turning pieces to coat all sides. Cover and refrigerate to marinate for 2 hours, turning every 20 minutes.

2. Preheat broiler.

3. Coat broiler rack with cooking spray. Place chicken on rack and broil about 6 inches from heat, turning to brown on all sides and brushing with marinade, for about 45 minutes or until chicken is brown, tender, and cooked through.

4. Transfer chicken to a heated platter, sprinkle with chopped cilantro, and serve.

SERVES 4

Per serving: 240 calories; 35.5 grams protein; 5.0 grams carbohydrates; 8.4 grams fat; 115 milligrams cholesterol; 130 milligrams sodium (without salting).

CHICKEN CUTLETS BROILED WITH TOMATOES AND MOZZARELLA

Serve this low fat version of Chicken Parmigiana with your favorite pasta and a salad of mixed crisp greens.

3/4 pound chicken cutlets, cut in 2-inch strips
2 teaspoons olive oil
1 tablespoon white wine vinegar
Salt and freshly ground pepper to taste
4 ripe plum tomatoes, seeded and chopped
1 teaspoon dried oregano
1 teaspoon dried parsley
1/4 teaspoon hot red pepper flakes or to taste, optional
1/2 cup canned low sodium tomato sauce
1 ounce shredded low fat mozzarella cheese

1. Place chicken in a medium bowl. Add oil, vinegar, and salt and pepper. Cover and refrigerate for 2 to 3 hours, turning chicken cutlets occasionally.

2. Preheat broiler.

3. Place tomatoes in a small saucepan. Add oregano, parsley, hot pepper flakes if desired, and tomato sauce. Bring to simmer and cook over medium-low heat for 10 minutes, stirring occasionally. Remove from heat.

4. Spoon about two-thirds of the tomato mixture from saucepan to bottom of a shallow ovenproof casserole. Top with chicken strips, then cover chicken

with remaining tomato mixture. Place about 5 inches from heat and broil for 15 minutes. Sprinkle cheese over chicken and tomatoes and broil for an additional 10 to 15 minutes or until chicken is cooked through and cheese is bubbly.

5. Remove from oven and serve immediately.

SERVES 4

Per serving: 160 calories; 22.5 grams protein; 7.5 grams carbohydrates; 4.5 grams fat; 51 milligrams cholesterol; 130 milligrams sodium (without salting).

SKEWERED CHICKEN WITH VEGETABLES IN APRICOT-MUSTARD MARINADE

Broiling is one of my favorite cooking methods for meats and chicken because it allows the fat to drain away. I use a broiler pan with a rack, which facilitates the process. And because I'm inherently lazy, I line the lower pan with foil for easy cleanup. Naturally this recipe works just as well on an outdoor grill.

1 cup apricot nectar
½ cup cranberry juice
2 teaspoons dry mustard
Salt and freshly ground pepper to taste
1 pound skinless and boneless chicken breasts, fat removed, cut into large chunks
1 large onion, quartered
4 large mushroom caps
1 medium green or red bell pepper, cut into 4 pieces
1 medium zucchini, cut into 4 pieces

1. Combine apricot nectar, cranberry juice, mustard, and salt and pepper in a small bowl and mix well. Transfer half of the apricot-cranberry juice mixture to a small serving bowl.

2. Place chicken in a medium bowl and spoon on remaining apricot-cranberry mixture, turning to coat chicken on all sides. Cover and let stand 20 minutes.

3. Prepare grill or preheat broiler.

4. Alternate chicken chunks and vegetables on skewers. Grill or broil about 5 inches from heat, turning skewers frequently to brown ingredients on all sides and brushing with leftover marinade, for 15 to 20 minutes or until chicken and vegetables are cooked through.

5. Transfer to a platter and serve with reserved sauce on the side.

SERVES 4

Per serving: 195 calories; 28.0 grams protein; 15.5 grams carbohydrates; 2.2 grams fat; 65 milligrams cholesterol; 80 milligrams sodium (without salting).

BROILED TURKEY BREAST
WITH HERB MARINADE

Although turkey has its own distinctive and, yes, delicate flavor, it is the perfect foil for ingredients that have a more pronounced taste. Like chicken, turkey is complemented by seasonings or herbs as assertive as sage, tarragon, and rosemary, as outlined in the recipe here. My relish, made with tomatoes, cucumbers, fresh parsley, and rice wine vinegar offers an excellent contrast.

  1 teaspoon dried sage
  1 teaspoon dried tarragon
  $1/2$ teaspoon dried marjoram
  $1/2$ teaspoon red pepper flakes
    Salt and freshly ground pepper to taste
  $1/2$ cup dry white wine
  2 teaspoons olive oil
  $1^1/2$ pounds skinless and boneless turkey breast, in one
    piece
    Vegetable oil cooking spray
  3 plum tomatoes, chopped
  2 cucumbers, peeled and chopped
  2 tablespoons chopped fresh parsley or basil
  1 tablespoon rice wine vinegar

1. Combine sage, tarragon, marjoram, red pepper flakes, salt and pepper, wine, and oil in a small bowl. Mix thoroughly. Place turkey in a shallow pan and pour herb marinade over turkey. Cover and refriger-

ate for 1 hour, turning turkey in marinade every 15 minutes.

2. Preheat broiler.

3. Place turkey in a broiler pan coated with cooking spray. Broil about 6 inches from heat, brushing occasionally with marinade, for 35 to 45 minutes or until tender and cooked through.

4. While turkey cooks, combine tomatoes, cucumbers, parsley or basil, and rice wine vinegar in a small serving bowl. Mix and set aside.

5. Remove cooked turkey from broiler and allow to rest 5 minutes. Cut turkey into thin slices and arrange on a serving platter. Spoon tomato combination over turkey and serve.

SERVES 6

Per serving: 170 calories; 29.0 grams protein; 6.5 grams carbohydrates; 3.3 grams fat; 71 milligrams cholesterol; 65 milligrams sodium (without salting).

TURKEY AND FRESH CORN KEBABS WITH PEPPER AND ONION

This dish can easily be cooked under a broiler, but grilling on hot coals makes these kebabs extra special.

1½ pounds skinless and boneless turkey breast, in one
    piece
  2 ears fresh corn, each cut crosswise into 6 pieces
  2 red bell peppers, each cut into 6 pieces
  1 large Spanish onion, cut in 6 wedges and separated
1½ tablespoons vegetable oil
    Juice from 2 limes
  1 tablespoon chili powder
  ¼ teaspoon cayenne pepper or to taste
    Salt to taste

1. Cut turkey into 1½-inch cubes and place in a deep bowl with corn, bell peppers, and onion.

2. Combine remaining ingredients in a small bowl and stir until well blended. Spoon mixture over turkey and vegetables and turn to coat on all sides. Let stand at room temperature for 30 minutes, turning turkey and vegetables occasionally.

3. Prepare grill.

4. Thread 6 metal skewers alternately with turkey, corn, red pepper, and onion pieces. Brush well with remaining marinade and grill 5 to 6 inches from coals

for about 15 minutes or until turkey and vegetables are cooked through, turning skewers to grill all sides.

SERVES 6
Per serving: 215 calories; 29.5 grams protein; 12.5 grams carbohydrates; 5.2 grams fat; 71 milligrams cholesterol; 75 milligrams sodium (without salting).

GRILLED TURKEY AND PINEAPPLE WITH DIPPING SAUCE

Pineapple serves as a vibrant compatriot for chicken when grilled (or broiled) with this sweet-and-sour marinade. The addictive dipping sauce will sneak up on you with its gentle explosion of heat. Serve with steamed basmati rice and crisp-steamed broccoli florets.

1/4 cup pineapple juice
1 tablespoon white wine vinegar
2 teaspoons vegetable or peanut oil
1 tablespoon dried crumbled mint
Salt and freshly ground pepper to taste
4 turkey breast cutlets (about 1 pound total)
1 ripe fresh pineapple, peeled, cored, and sliced into 4 thick rings

DIPPING SAUCE
3/4 cup pineapple juice
1/4 cup rice or white wine vinegar
1 teaspoon dried crumbled mint
2 teaspoons low sodium soy sauce
1/2 teaspoon hot sesame oil or chili paste, or to taste

1. Combine 1/4 cup pineapple juice with vinegar, oil, mint, and salt and pepper in a small bowl. Stir to blend thoroughly.

2. Place turkey cutlets and pineapple slices in a large

bowl. Spoon pineapple-vinegar mixture over turkey and pineapple, covering all sides. Cover bowl and refrigerate for 30 minutes to 1 hour.

3. Prepare grill or preheat broiler.

4. Prepare dipping sauce by combining all ingredients in a food processor and process until smoothly blended. Transfer to a small bowl and let stand at room temperature until needed.

5. Grill or broil turkey 5 to 6 inches from heat, turning once, for about 6 minutes on each side or until turkey is cooked through. Add pineapple slices and grill on both sides halfway during grilling turkey.

6. Transfer turkey and pineapple to a heated serving platter and serve with dipping sauce on the side.

SERVES 4

Per serving: 185 calories; 28.5 grams protein; 7.5 grams carbohydrates; 4.1 grams fat; 71 milligrams cholesterol; 160 milligrams sodium (without salting).

THE MAIN DISH:
STEWED AND POACHED

SOUTHERN-STYLE
CHICKEN-OKRA STEW

I first fell in love with okra in New Orleans where it is cooked in every manner you can imagine. I dote on its flavor, and I even adore the curious property that causes okra to exude a sticky juice when cut and cooked that some folks dislike. Southern cooks use this quality to their advantage so beautifully. The mucilage-like material behaves in much the same way as cornstarch, thus the surprising okra will thicken and give body to any liquid to which it is added.

Nutritionally, this wonder-pod is a good source of vitamin C and dietary fiber, yet it's extremely low in calories, fat, and sodium.

When you sample my chicken-okra stew, you, too, will be a die-hard okraholic. Serve with rice.

1 teaspoon olive oil
1 large onion, chopped
1 pound skinless and boneless chicken breasts, fat
    removed, cubed
4 medium ripe tomatoes, peeled and chopped
2 cups Low Fat Chicken Stock (page 3) or canned low
    sodium broth
1 bay leaf
1/2 teaspoon dried thyme
1/2 teaspoon chili powder or to taste

³⁄₄ pound young okra, trimmed and cut into ¹⁄₄-inch
    pieces
    Salt and freshly ground pepper to taste

1. Heat oil in a soup pot or Dutch oven. Add onion and chicken and cook over medium-high heat, stirring, for 3 minutes.

2. Add tomatoes, stock, bay leaf, thyme, and chili powder. Bring to a slow simmer, cover, and cook for 30 minutes.

3. Add okra and cook for an additional 15 minutes or until okra and chicken are tender.

4. Taste and add salt and pepper or correct seasonings, if necessary. Discard bay leaf before serving.

SERVES 4

Per serving: 225 calories; 30.0 grams protein; 17.5 grams carbohydrates; 4.0 grams fat; 67 milligrams cholesterol; 130 milligrams sodium (without salting).

CHICKEN RAGOUT WITH ENDIVE

A "ragout" is a thick, well-seasoned stew of meat, poultry, or fish that is made either with or without vegetables. In this easy-to-do recipe, I've combined endive with chicken thighs for a heartier taste, and added a combination of dried herbs you probably already have stocked in your pantry.

When eaten raw in salads, endive has a pleasantly bitter taste. Braising will tame its bite while mellowing its flavor.

1 teaspoon olive oil
4 chicken thighs (about 1 pound total), skin and fat removed
Salt and freshly ground pepper to taste
4 Belgian endives
2 cups Low Fat Chicken Stock (page 3) or canned low sodium broth
Juice of 1/2 lemon
1 teaspoon herbes de Provence, or 1/4 teaspoon each: dried thyme, marjoram, rosemary, sage

1. Heat oil in a large skillet or Dutch oven. Add chicken and season with salt and pepper. Cook over medium-high heat for 2 minutes on each side or until chicken is lightly browned but not cooked through.

2. Place endive beside chicken and add all remaining ingredients. Cover and cook over low heat for 30 to 40 minutes or until chicken is tender and cooked through.

3. Transfer chicken and endive to a heated platter, pour sauce over all, and serve hot.

SERVES 4

Per serving: 150 calories; 17.0 grams protein; 10.0 grams carbohydrates; 5.2 grams fat; 60 milligrams cholesterol; 150 milligrams sodium (without salting).

RAGOUT OF CHICKEN
WITH OREGANO AND WINE

Oregano is another one of those elusive herbs that will taste as good in its fresh or dried state, and I always have a jar stored in a cool, dark place where it keeps for up to six months.

This pungent herb is a member of the mint family and is related to both marjoram and thyme. Although oregano is the indispensable flavoring on pizza, it is most prevalent in Greek cuisine. The recipe below was inspired by a dish I enjoyed at a taverna on the island of Corfu some years ago.

1 3-pound chicken, skin and fat removed, quartered
2 stalks celery, thinly sliced
4 shallots, minced
1/2 teaspoon oregano or to taste
   Salt and freshly ground pepper to taste
1/4 teaspoon hot pepper flakes or to taste, optional
1/2 cup dry white wine
1/2 cup low sodium tomato juice

1. Place chicken in a soup pot or Dutch oven. Strew celery and shallots around chicken and sprinkle with oregano, salt and pepper, and hot pepper flakes if desired.

2. Combine wine and tomato juice in a small bowl and pour over chicken. Cover and cook over low heat for 45 minutes to 1 hour or until chicken is tender and cooked through.

3. Using a slotted spoon, remove chicken to a platter and keep warm.

4. Simmer sauce in pot until reduced by about one-third and spoon over chicken before serving.

SERVES 4
Per serving: 220 calories; 36.0 grams protein; 6.0 grams carbohydrates; 5.3 grams fat; 115 milligrams cholesterol; 150 milligrams sodium (without salting).

CHICKEN STEWED WITH PEAS AND POTATOES IN CIDER

This hearty and wholesome one-pot meal needs nothing save for a glistening salad of greens and some good crusty Italian bread.

1 teaspoon vegetable oil
1 small onion, minced
1 clove garlic, pressed
1 3-pound chicken, skin and fat removed, cut into 8 pieces
1 cup Low Fat Chicken Stock (page 3) or canned low sodium broth
1 cup apple juice or cider
1 tablespoon cider vinegar
2 medium potatoes, peeled and cut into small cubes
2 cups fresh or frozen green peas
Salt and freshly ground pepper to taste

1. Heat oil in a large nonstick skillet or soup pot. Add chicken and sauté until chicken is golden on all sides. Add onion and garlic and stir over medium heat for 1 minute.

2. Add stock, cider or juice, and vinegar and bring to a simmer. Cover and cook over medium-low heat for 20 minutes.

3. Add potatoes and cook an additional 15 minutes.

4. Reduce heat to low, add peas and salt and pepper to taste. Simmer gently, uncovered, for 10 minutes or until chicken and potato are cooked through.

Per serving: 315 calories; 39.0 grams protein; 23.5 grams carbohydrates; 7.0 grams fat; 117 milligrams cholesterol; 155 milligrams sodium (without salting).

HUNGARIAN CHICKEN PAPRIKA

Classically, this Hungarian standby is made by browning skin-on chicken and onions in bacon drippings and topped with a sauce consisting of the cooking liquid mixed with sour cream. Chicken skin? Bacon drippings? Sour cream? Definite no-nos!

In my slimmed-down version, I use just two teaspoons of olive oil. The sauce is made with the cooking liquid and low fat yogurt, losing nothing but extra fat in the translation.

Serve this delicious dish in the traditional fashion, with plain broad noodles.

2 teaspoons olive oil
1 3-pound chicken, skin and fat removed, cut into 8
    pieces
1 small onion, finely chopped
2 cloves garlic, pressed
1 teaspoon sweet paprika
    Pinch hot paprika or to taste
1/2 cup Low Fat Chicken Stock (page 3) or canned low
    sodium broth
1/2 cup low fat plain yogurt
    Salt to taste
1 tablespoon chopped fresh parsley

1. Heat oil in a soup pot or Dutch oven. Cook chicken over medium-high heat for about 5 minutes or until lightly browned on all sides.

2. Add onion, garlic, sweet and hot paprika, and chicken stock to pot. Cover and simmer over medium heat for 45 minutes to 1 hour or until chicken is tender.

3. Stir in yogurt and add salt to taste. Bring to a simmer and cook, covered, for 5 minutes.

4. Spoon chicken with sauce into a deep serving platter. Garnish with parsley and serve hot.

SERVES 4

Per serving: 245 calories; 37.5 grams protein; 5.0 grams carbohydrates; 8.2 grams fat; 117 milligrams cholesterol; 160 milligrams sodium (without salting).

CHICKEN MOLE

Chicken with chocolate? This Mexican dish proves that the combination really works. Chocolate was originally cultivated in Mexico, and the small amount used in this recipe adds just the right touch to this exotic stew. For an authentic touch, serve with corn tortillas.

1 teaspoon olive oil
1 3-pound chicken, skin and fat removed, cut into 8 pieces
  Salt and freshly ground pepper to taste
2 cups Low Fat Chicken Stock (page 3) or canned low sodium broth
1/2 teaspoon fennel seeds
1 teaspoon sesame seeds
2 cloves garlic
1/4 teaspoon dried coriander
  Pinch ground cloves
1 teaspoon golden raisins
1/2 ounce unsweetened bitter chocolate, grated
2 ripe tomatoes, halved
1 jalapeño pepper, cored and seeded

1. Heat oil in a Dutch oven or a deep nonstick skillet with a lid. Season chicken and sauté over medium-high heat for about 5 minutes or until chicken is lightly brown on all sides. Remove from heat.

2. Combine all remaining ingredients in a food

processor or blender and process until sauce is smooth.

3. Pour sauce over chicken in pot and bring to a simmer. Cover and cook over low heat for about 1 hour or until the sauce has been partially absorbed by the chicken, and chicken is tender.

SERVES 6
Per serving: 185 calories; 24.5 grams protein; 7.0 grams carbohydrates; 6.4 grams fat; 79 milligrams cholesterol; 155 milligrams sodium (without salting).

CHICKEN WITH POLENTA, TOMATOES, AND CORN

Polenta is cornmeal, and this recipe calls for cornmeal and corn kernels, a double delight for corn lovers. This is really a great party dish. It can be prepared in advance up to the final baking, and since only a fork is required it's easy to eat while moving around a house or patio.

1 whole chicken breast (about 1 pound), skin and fat
    removed
5 cups water
1 medium onion, cut in half
1 bay leaf
1 celery stalk, cut in half
1 carrot, cut in half
    Salt and freshly ground pepper to taste
1/2 cup yellow cornmeal
1 cup chopped onion
2 cloves garlic, pressed
4 plum tomatoes, chopped
1 teaspoon chili powder or to taste
1 1/2 cups fresh or frozen and thawed corn kernels
    Vegetable oil cooking spray

1. In a soup pot or Dutch oven, combine chicken, water, onion, bay leaf, celery, carrot, and salt and pepper to taste. Bring to a boil, then cover and reduce to a simmer. Cook for about 30 minutes or until

chicken is tender and cooked through. Remove chicken from broth and set aside to cool.

2. Strain broth, reserving 2 cups, and discard solids.

3. To make polenta, heat 1 1/2 cups of reserved broth in a small saucepan and bring to a boil. Add cornmeal gradually and cook at a simmer, stirring frequently, for 10 to 20 minutes or until polenta thickens. Remove from heat and set aside.

4. Preheat oven to 350° F.

5. Combine remaining 1/2 cup broth with chopped onion, garlic, and tomatoes in a small saucepan. Simmer over medium-low heat, stirring occasionally, for 10 minutes. Add chili powder and corn and cook for an additional minute.

6. Cut chicken away from bone and cube. Discard bones.

7. To assemble dish, spread polenta on the bottom of an ovenproof casserole lightly coated with cooking spray. Top with cubed chicken and cover with tomato-corn mixture.

8. Bake for 30 minutes. Bring casserole to the table and serve immediately.

SERVES 4

Per serving: 230 calories; 18.0 grams protein; 32.5 grams carbohydrates; 3.2 grams fat; 32 milligrams cholesterol; 270 milligrams sodium (without salting).

FRICASSEE OF CHICKEN WITH SHRIMP AND TURKEY SAUSAGE

Poultry and shrimp have long been eaten together in Chinese, Portuguese, and Spanish cuisines, and this easy-to-assemble recipe will point up their complementary features.

Potatoes, rice, orzo, or a thin pasta would go extremely well with this splendid dish.

1 teaspoon olive oil
1/2 skinless and boneless chicken breast (about 1/2 pound), cut into 4 pieces
1 red bell pepper, cut into strips
2 tomatoes, quartered
1/4 pound Italian turkey sausage, thinly sliced
Salt and freshly ground pepper to taste
1 bay leaf
1 1/2 cups Low Fat Chicken Stock (page 3) or canned low sodium broth
1/2 cup dry white wine
1/4 pound medium shrimp, shelled, deveined, and rinsed

1. Heat oil in a soup pot or Dutch oven. Add chicken and cook over medium-high heat for 2 minutes on each side or until golden.

2. Add bell pepper and tomatoes and cook for 1 minute. Add sausage and cook, stirring, for another minute.

3. Add all remaining ingredients, except shrimp, and reduce heat to low. Cover and cook, stirring occa-

sionally, for 15 minutes. Add shrimp and cook, uncovered, for an additional 5 minutes.

4. Remove bay leaf, transfer to a heated platter, and
serve hot.

SERVES 4

Per serving: 195 calories; 24.5 grams protein; 8.5 grams
carbohydrates; 7.3 grams fat; 107 milligrams cholesterol;
300 milligrams sodium (without salting).

CHICKEN AND RICE
WITH PARSLEY-MINT SAUCE

The combination of parsley and mint casts a magnificent emerald hue over the chicken and rice and imparts a very different flavor. I'd opt to serve a vegetable or salad with a decided color contrast as an accompaniment—sliced, dead-ripe tomatoes, for example.

2 teaspoons olive oil
1 3-pound chicken, skin and fat removed, cut into 8
    pieces
  Salt and freshly ground pepper to taste
1 cup rice
1/2 cup packed fresh parsley
1/4 cup packed fresh mint or 2 tablespoons dried
1 large onion, cut in pieces
2 cups Low Fat Chicken Stock (page 3) or canned low
    sodium broth, approximate
1 lemon cut into wedges

1. Heat oil in a nonstick soup pot or Dutch oven. Add chicken pieces in one layer and cook over high heat for about 5 minutes or until lightly browned on all sides. Do not cook chicken through. Remove from pot, season to taste, and set aside.

2. Add rice to pot and cook, stirring, for 1 or 2 minutes or until rice is no longer translucent. Add chicken to rice in pot and remove from heat.

3. Combine parsley, mint, onion, and 1 cup stock in

a food processor and process until ingredients are pureed. Combine with remaining stock and stir until well-blended.

4. Pour parsley-stock mixture over chicken and rice. Cover and cook over low heat for 30 to 45 minutes or until chicken and rice are completely cooked, adding additional stock or water if necessary. Transfer chicken and rice to a heated platter and serve garnished with lemon wedges.

SERVES 4

Per serving: 420 calories; 40.0 grams protein; 44.5 grams carbohydrates; 8.8 grams fat; 118 milligrams cholesterol; 170 milligrams sodium (without salting).

RAGOUT OF TURKEY
WITH FENNEL

I happen to be a freak for fennel! I love its mild, aniselike flavor when cooked. If you do not yet share my fanaticism for *finocchio*, I believe that this recipe will make you a convert.

>   2 teaspoons olive oil
>   2 tablespoons dry vermouth
>   2 cups Low Fat Chicken Stock (page 3) or canned low
>   sodium broth
>   2 cloves garlic, pressed
>   1/2 teaspoon freshly ground pepper
>   Salt to taste
>   8 turkey breast cutlets (about 1 pound total)
>   1 large fennel bulb, thinly sliced

1. Combine 1 teaspoon olive oil, vermouth, 1/2 cup stock, garlic, pepper and salt in a small bowl. Mix well.

2. Place turkey in a shallow pan. Pour oil-vermouth combination over turkey, turn in marinade to coat all sides. Refrigerate for 1 hour, turning turkey in marinade every 15 minutes.

3. Remove turkey from marinade and scrape marinade from turkey. Set aside turkey and marinade.

4. Heat remaining teaspoon oil in a soup pot or Dutch oven. Sauté turkey over medium-high heat for 2 minutes on each side or until lightly browned. Remove turkey and set aside. Add reserved marinade

and remainder of stock to pot. Bring to a simmer and add fennel. Cover and cook until fennel is almost tender, about 15 minutes.

5. Return turkey to pot. Cover and cook an additional 5 to 10 minutes, or until turkey and fennel are tender.

6. Place turkey cutlets on a heated platter or individual plates, spoon fennel and sauce over cutlets, and serve.

SERVES 4

Per serving: 180 calories; 29.0 grams protein; 6.5 grams carbohydrates; 4.2 grams fat; 74 milligrams cholesterol; 120 milligrams sodium (without salting).

CURRIED TURKEY AND BABY CARROTS IN YOGURT SAUCE

Here, seasoned yogurt does double duty as the marinade and cooking medium for turkey and baby carrots. Couple it with fragrant basmati or texmati rice, or minted lentils.

> 1 pound skinless and boneless turkey breast, cut into 1-inch squares
> 1/2 cup low fat plain yogurt
> 1 clove garlic, pressed
> 1 tablespoon chopped fresh coriander leaves (cilantro) or 1/2 tablespoon dried
> 1/2 teaspoon freshly ground pepper
> 1/2 tablespoon vegetable oil
> 1 small onion, finely chopped
> 1 cup whole tiny baby carrots, or small baby carrots cut in half lengthwise
> 1 1/2 cups Low Fat Chicken Stock (page 3) or canned low sodium broth
> 1 tablespoon curry powder, or to taste
> 1/2 teaspoon dried cardamom
> Salt to taste
> Chopped fresh coriander leaves (cilantro) for garnish

1. Combine turkey, yogurt, garlic, coriander, and pepper in a medium bowl. Mix well and refrigerate for 1 hour, turning occasionally.

---

2. Heat oil in a Dutch oven or casserole. Add onion, and cook, stirring for 1 minute.

3. Add turkey with marinade, carrots, stock, and curry powder to Dutch oven. Stir to combine.

4. Cover and simmer for 15 minutes or until turkey and carrots are tender. Serve garnished with fresh coriander leaves.

SERVES 4

Per serving: 195 calories; 30.5 grams protein; 9.0 grams carbohydrates; 4.0 grams fat; 75 milligrams cholesterol; 135 milligrams sodium (without salting).

CHUNKY TURKEY CHILI

This is a real crowd pleaser; just don't be turned off by the number of ingredients involved. With the exception of one or two fresh items, you probably have most of them in your kitchen already.

Serve with heated pita triangles or corn tortillas.

2 teaspoons vegetable oil
1 large onion, chopped
1 green bell pepper, chopped
2 cloves garlic, chopped
1 small hot chili pepper, seeded and minced, or
   1 teaspoon hot pepper flakes
1 28-ounce can low sodium peeled tomatoes, with juice,
   coarsely chopped
1 cup canned no-salt-added tomato sauce
1/2 cup red table wine
2 tablespoons chopped fresh coriander leaves (cilantro)
   or parsley
1 1/2 tablespoons chili powder or to taste
1 teaspoon dried oregano
1 teaspoon ground cumin
   Salt to taste
1 1/2 pounds skinless and boneless turkey breast or thighs,
   cut into 1 1/2-inch cubes
2 cups cooked red kidney beans or canned (rinsed and
   drained)
2 tablespoons low fat sour cream
2 tablespoons finely minced red onions

1. Heat oil in a soup pot or Dutch oven. Add onion and stir over medium-low heat for 5 minutes or until softened. Add bell pepper, garlic, and chili pepper and stir for 1 minute.

2. Add tomatoes, tomato sauce, and wine and bring to a boil. Reduce heat to medium and stir in coriander, chili powder, oregano, cumin, and salt to taste. Let simmer 5 minutes. Reduce heat to low, cover, and simmer gently, stirring occasionally, for 20 minutes.

3. Add turkey and beans to pot. Taste and adjust seasonings, if necessary, and stir to blend. Continue to cook, covered, for an additional 15 to 20 minutes or until turkey is cooked through.

4. Ladle into heated bowls and sprinkle each serving with 1 teaspoon of red onions and 1 teaspoon of sour cream. Serve hot.

SERVES 6

Per serving: 290 calories; 35.0 grams protein; 29.0 grams carbohydrates; 4.4 grams fat; 73 milligrams cholesterol; 220 milligrams sodium (without salting).

RED CABBAGE TURKEY ROLLS
IN TOMATO-WINE SAUCE

The robust flavors of red cabbage and turkey sausage combine with a rich tomato-wine sauce to make this delicious dish truly memorable.

> 1 medium head red cabbage (about 1³/₄ pounds)
> 1 pound mild Italian turkey sausage, casings removed, or plain ground turkey
> 1 onion, grated or finely minced
> 2 cloves garlic, finely minced
> 2 tablespoons chopped fresh parsley
> 1 teaspoon dried oregano
>   Salt and freshly ground pepper to taste
>   Egg substitute equal to 1 egg
> 1 28-ounce can low sodium crushed tomatoes
> 1 cup Burgundy or other full-bodied dry red wine
> 1 cup water, approximately

1. Core cabbage and place in a large pot with enough water to nearly cover. Cover and bring to a boil. Cook for about 5 minutes or until leaves are soft. Drain well and let cool slightly. Carefully remove the outer 12 leaves and set aside. Shred remaining cabbage and set aside.

2. In a large bowl, combine turkey sausage with onion, garlic, parsley, oregano, salt and pepper. Mix well. Add egg substitute and mix again until ingredients are thoroughly combined.

3. Separate turkey mixture into 12 balls and place a

ball in center of each cabbage leaf. Fold in sides and roll up each leaf. As they are rolled, place each leaf, seam-side down in a large pot. Place rolls close together and stack, if necessary.

4. Add shredded cabbage and tomatoes to pot, then pour in wine and water. Cabbage rolls should be just covered with liquid; if not, add additional water. Bring to a boil, then reduce heat to very low, cover, and let simmer gently for 1 hour, adding additional water or wine if too much liquid evaporates.

5. Spoon rolls with shredded cabbage and sauce onto a deep platter and serve hot.

SERVES 6

Per serving: 245 calories; 17.0 grams protein; 22.0 grams carbohydrates; 10.3 grams fat; 80 milligrams cholesterol; 550 milligrams sodium (without salting).

TURKEY TONNATO

Traditionally made with veal and served chilled and thinly sliced, this Italian dish is equally good hot or at room temperature. However you serve it, turkey in tuna sauce is a dish everyone seems to love.

½ skinless and boneless turkey breast (about 1¾ pounds), rolled and tied
1 6⅛-ounce can water-packed low sodium tuna
1 large onion, chopped
1 stalk celery, chopped
1 carrot, chopped
2 cloves garlic, quartered
4 anchovies, rinsed and diced
1 tablespoon minced fresh parsley or ½ tablespoon dried
1 teaspoon dried thyme
2 cups water
1 cup dry white wine
1 cup low fat plain yogurt
2 tablespoons fresh lemon juice
2 tablespoons capers, rinsed and drained
Salt and freshly ground pepper to taste
Lemon wedges and parsley sprigs for garnish

1. Roll turkey breast and secure in several places with kitchen string. Set aside.

2. In a large pot, combine tuna, onion, celery, carrot, garlic, anchovies, parsley, thyme, water, and wine. Bring to a boil, then reduce heat to very low.

Cover and simmer gently, stirring occasionally, for 30 minutes.

3. Add turkey to pot and continue cooking on low heat, covered, for an additional 30 minutes. Raise heat to medium, uncover, and cook for 20 minutes or until turkey is cooked through and liquid is reduced. Remove pot from heat, cover, and let stand until cool. Refrigerate the entire pot with its contents overnight or for at least 3 hours to chill well.

4. Remove turkey from pot and transfer to a cutting board. Cut off and discard strings.

5. Transfer sauce from pot to a food processor and process until coarsely pureed. Add yogurt, lemon juice, and salt and pepper to taste, and process until well blended. Transfer sauce to a mixing bowl and stir in capers.

6. Cut turkey into very thin slices. Arrange slices on a serving platter, overlapping them slightly. Spoon about ¾ cup of the sauce down center of turkey slices. Garnish platter with lemon wedges and parsley sprigs and serve remaining sauce on the side.

SERVES 8

Per serving: 175 calories; 32.5 grams protein; 7.5 grams carbohydrates; 1.5 grams fat; 72 milligrams cholesterol; 135 milligrams sodium (without salting).

INDEX